Human Anatomy Coloring Book

J. A. Gosling MD, MB, ChB, FRCS
Professor of Anatomy
Chinese University of Hong Kong
Hong Kong

P. F. Harris MD, MB, ChB, MSc
Professor and Head of Department
of Human and Clinical Anatomy
Sultan Qaboos University
Sultanate of Oman

J. R. Humpherson MB, ChB
Senior Lecturer in Anatomy
School of Biological Sciences
University of Manchester
United Kingdom

I. Whitmore MD, MB, BS, LRCP, MRCS
Senior Lecturer in Anatomy
Department of Anatomy
Queen Mary and Westfield College
London
United Kingdom

P. L. T. Willan MB, ChB, FRCS
Professor of Anatomy
University of UAE, Al-Ain
United Arab Emirates

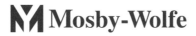

Mosby-Wolfe

London Baltimore Barcelona Bogotá Boston Buenos Aires Carlsbad, CA Chicago Madrid Mexico City Milan Naples, FL New York Philadelphia
St Louis Seoul Singapore Sydney Taipei Tokyo Toronto Wiesbaden

Publisher: Dianne Zack

Development editor: Louise Crowe

Project manager: Leslie Sinoway

Production: Gudrun Hughes

Design: Greg Smith

Cover design: Greg Smith

Cover photography: Alex Foreman

Illustration: Mike Saiz
                          Mark Willey
                          Lynda Payne
                          Lee Smith

Published in 1997 by Mosby–Wolfe, an imprint of Times Mirror International Publishers Limited

Printed by Vincenzo Bona, s.r.l, Turin.

ISBN 0 7234 2919 7

For full details of all Times Mirror International Publishers Limited titles, please write to Times Mirror International Publishers Limited, Lynton House, 7–12 Tavistock Square, London WC1H 9LB, England.

A CIP catalogue record for this book is available from the British Library.

Preface

The *Human Anatomy Coloring Book* was conceived as an extension of *Human Anatomy, Color Atlas and Text*, Third Edition by Gosling, Harris, Humpherson, Whitmore and Willan. In the preface to the First Edition of the *Color Atlas and Text* (1985), we noted 'this volume aims to provide the students with a better understanding of human anatomy'. Our aspirations have not changed.

The *Human Anatomy Coloring Book* contains line drawings, most of which are accurate anatomical drawings of dissections, the remainder being diagrammatic illustrations. Students should identify, colour and label the indicated components of the drawings. Checking the answers and correcting errors is essential. We know that such active participation in the educational process assists memory and subsequent understanding. We believe that the book provides a valuable self-test aid which will help students to recognise and remember specific anatomical structures and their relationships. In addition, it will support a typical anatomical text or colour atlas.

The authors are grateful to the team at Mosby–Wolfe in London UK who have had to cope with five authors located on three different continents and at five sites.

J.A.G., P.F.H., J.R.H., I.W., & P.L.T.W.
September, 1996

Contents

User Guide

This user guide explains how to use the colouring book. It is followed by eight chapters, each dealing with one of the following anatomical regions:

- basic anatomical systems
- thorax
- upper limb
- abdomen
- pelvis and perineum
- lower limb
- head and neck
- back

You should study each drawing carefully before starting to label and colour.

Leader lines

Most of the leader lines have been left unlabelled for you to fill in on identifying the structure. The leader lines are numbered and the correct answer to each is given in the Answer section at the back of the book.

Colouring notes

To make the most of colouring the drawings, you will need at least 12 different colours. You should always use red for arteries, blue for veins, yellow for nerves and brown for muscle. Light colours are better as dark colours may obscure detail. For best results, use coloured pencils with sharpened points. Wax crayons may not give lines fine enough for the level of detail required and felt tip pens may bleed through the paper. Select one colour for each of the following, and colour the box next to each so you can refer back to this table later:

☐	Artery		☐	Vein
☐	Nerve		☐	Muscle
☐	Mesentery		☐	Bone
☐	Fat		☐	Capsule
☐	Hyaline cartilage		☐	Fibrocartilage
☐	Organ		☐	Ligament
☐	Gland		☐	Duct

If you have a copy of Gosling *et al.*, *Human Anatomy Color Atlas and Text*, you may find it helpful to use the same colours that appear throughout the atlas, and then you can refer to the figures in the atlas to check you have coloured yours correctly. As a check that you have coloured the figures correctly, refer to the Answer section at the back of the book where the labels to each figure are given.

Orientation guides

Each figure is accompanied by an orientation guide whose axes use the following abbreviations:

L	left		**A**	anterior
R	right		**la**	lateral
S	superior		**m**	medial
I	inferior		**pr**	proximal
P	posterior		**d**	distal

Orientation guides in oblique views use large and small arrow heads and long and short arrow shafts. The following examples illustrate how orientation guides are used with the drawings in this book.

From in front

 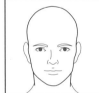

From behind

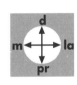 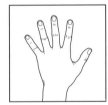

From the left side and slightly in front

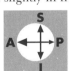 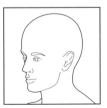

From the left side, slightly above and in front

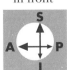 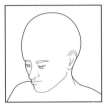

1. Basic Anatomical Systems

Fig. 1.1 Anterior view of the skeleton

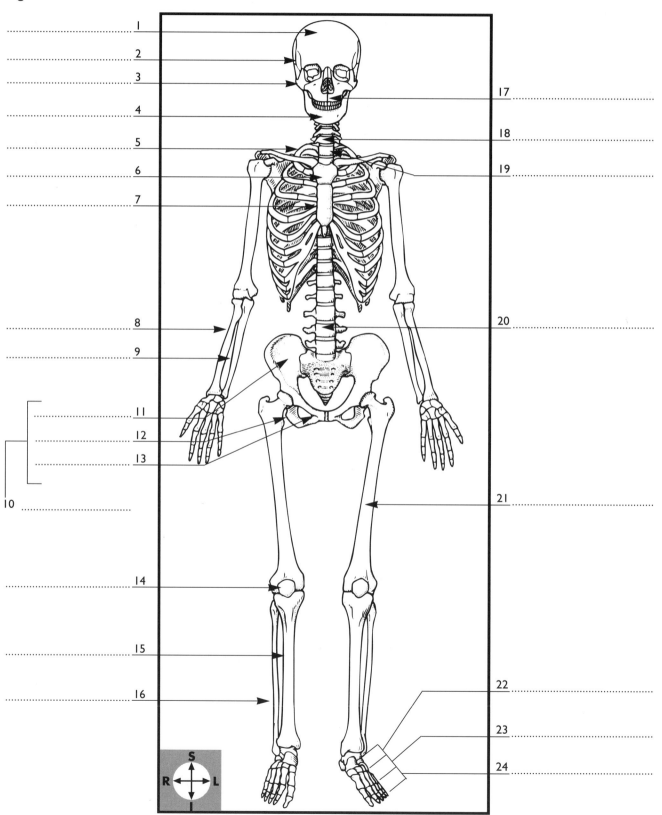

1 ....

2 ....

3 ....

4 ....

5 ....

6 ....

7 ....

8 ....

9 ....

11 ....

12 ....

13 ....

10 ....

14 ....

15 ....

16 ....

17 ....

18 ....

19 ....

20 ....

21 ....

22 ....

23 ....

24 ....

Fig. 1.2 Posterior view of the skeleton

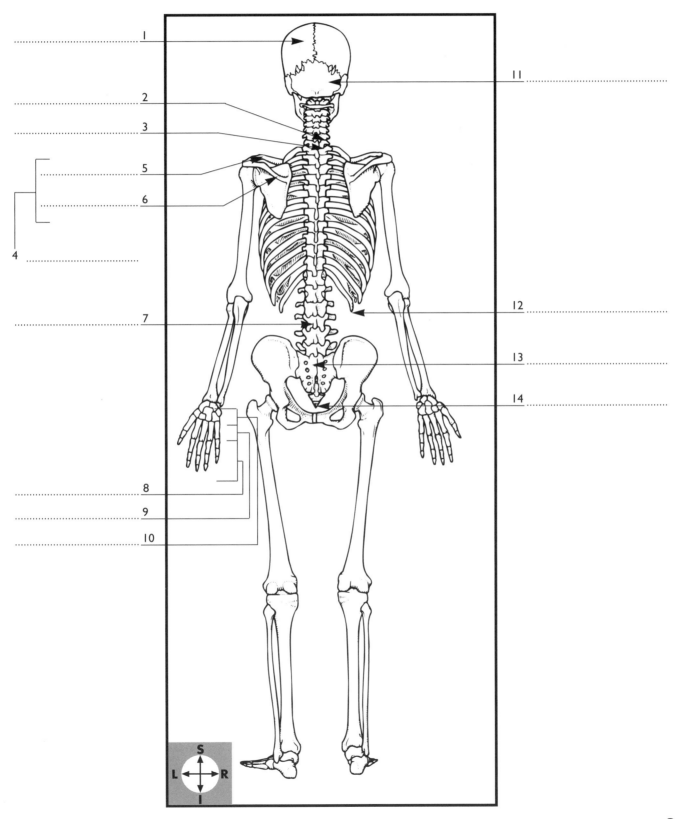

Fig. 1.3 Principal systemic arteries

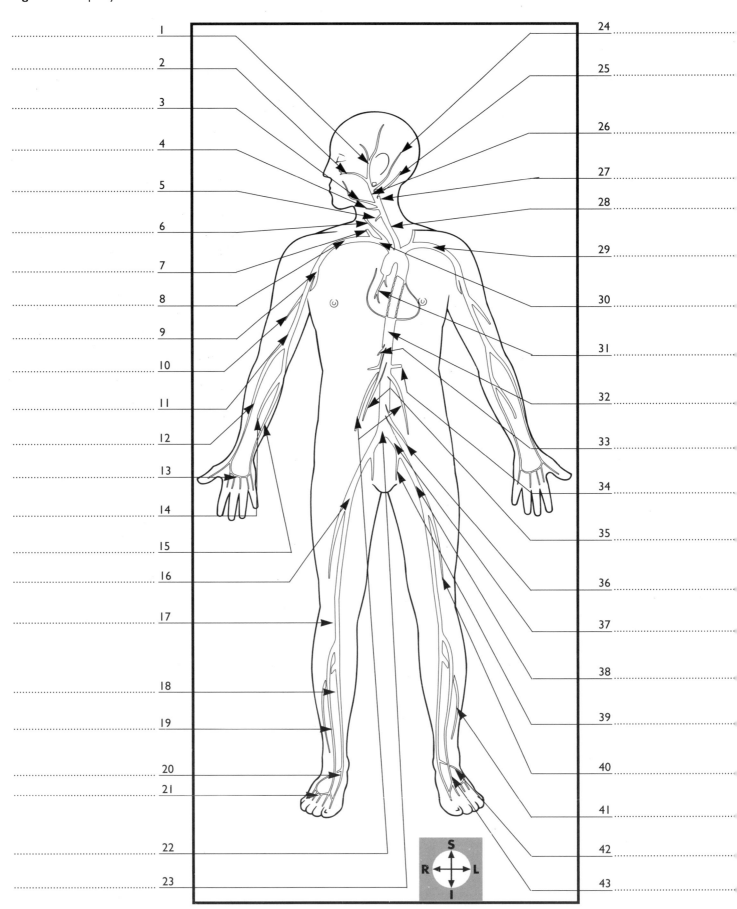

1 ....
2 ....
3 ....
4 ....
5 ....
6 ....
7 ....
8 ....
9 ....
10 ....
11 ....
12 ....
13 ....
14 ....
15 ....
16 ....
17 ....
18 ....
19 ....
20 ....
21 ....
22 ....
23 ....

24 ....
25 ....
26 ....
27 ....
28 ....
29 ....
30 ....
31 ....
32 ....
33 ....
34 ....
35 ....
36 ....
37 ....
38 ....
39 ....
40 ....
41 ....
42 ....
43 ....

Fig. 1.4 Principal systemic veins

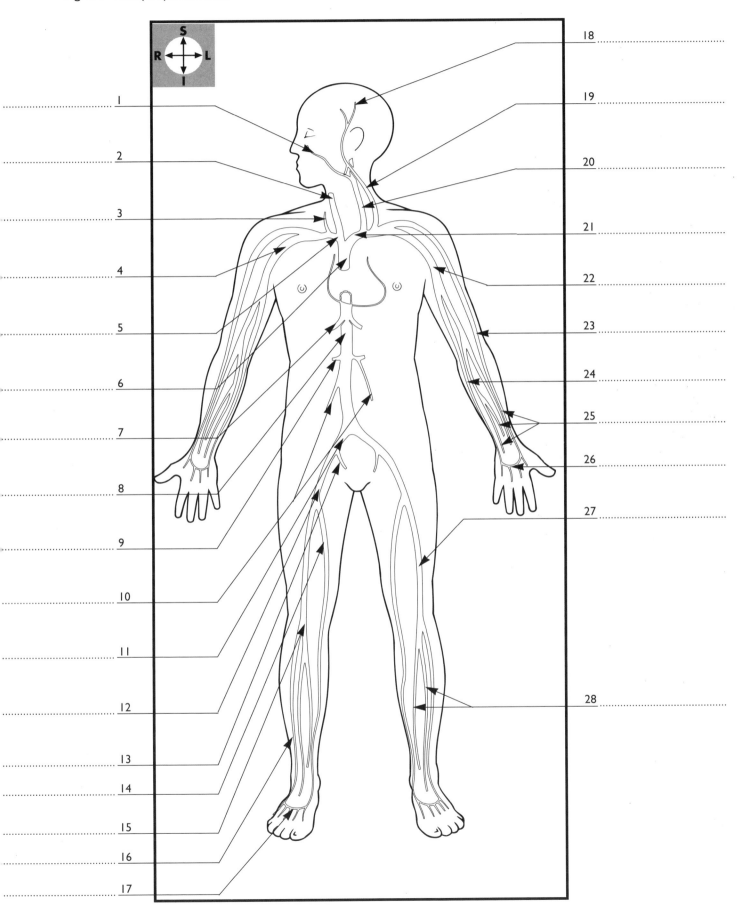

Fig. 1.5 Distribution of the anterior rami of the spinal nerves

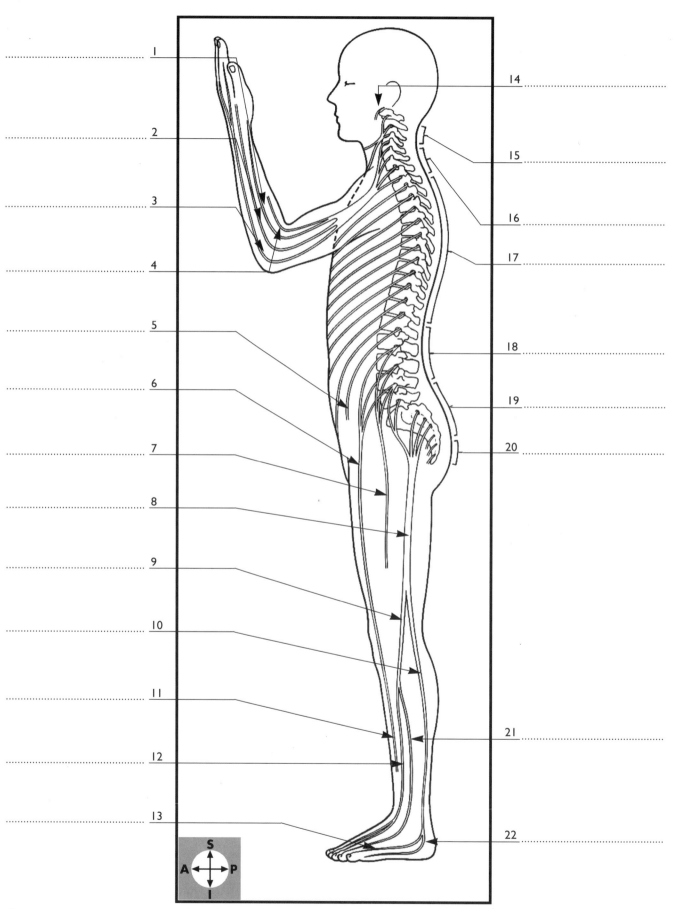

2. Thorax

Fig. 2.1 Articulated bones of the thorax showing the relationship between the vertebral column, ribs, costal cartilages and sternum

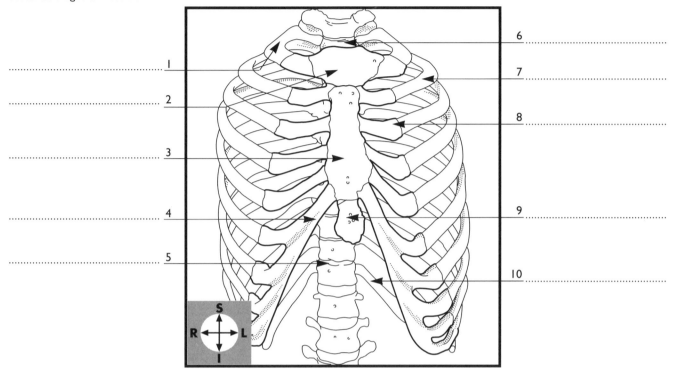

Fig. 2.2 Innermost intercostal muscles and intercostal nerves exposed after removing parts of the internal intercostal muscles. In the third intercostal space the innermost intercostal muscle has been removed to expose the parietal pleura

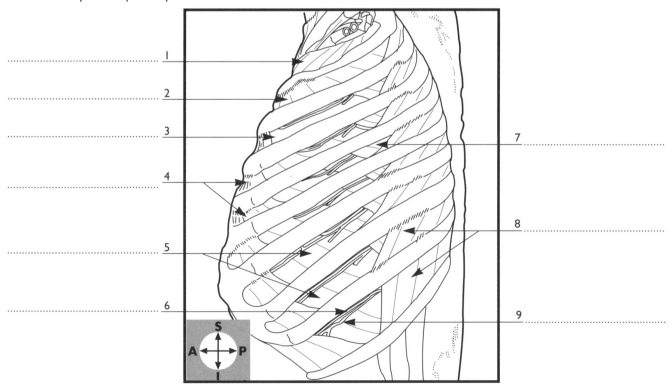

Fig. 2.3 Removal of the anterior chest wall has exposed the internal thoracic vessels and the costal part of the parietal pleura, through which the lungs are visible

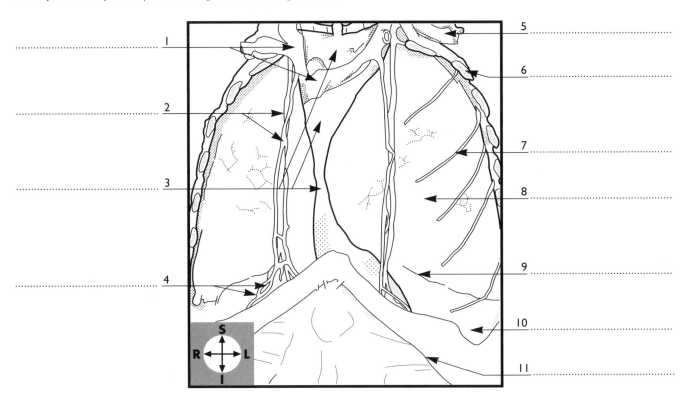

Fig. 2.4 Lungs after removal of the anterolateral thoracic wall and parietal pleura

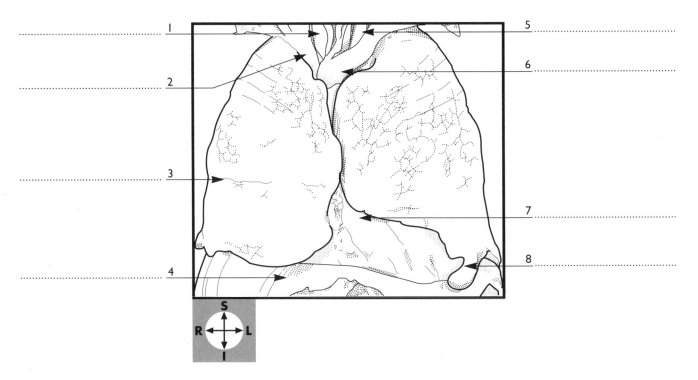

Fig. 2.5 The fibrous pericardium has been opened to expose the visceral pericardium covering the anterior surface of the heart

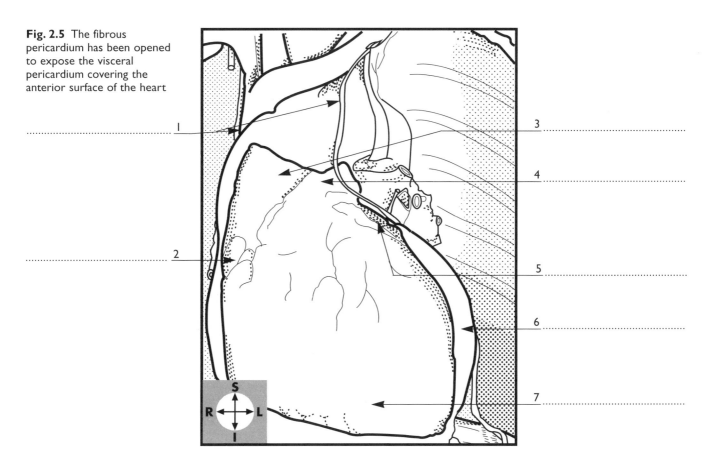

Fig. 2.6 Interior of the right atrium and atrial appendage exposed by reflection and excision of part of the anterior atrial wall

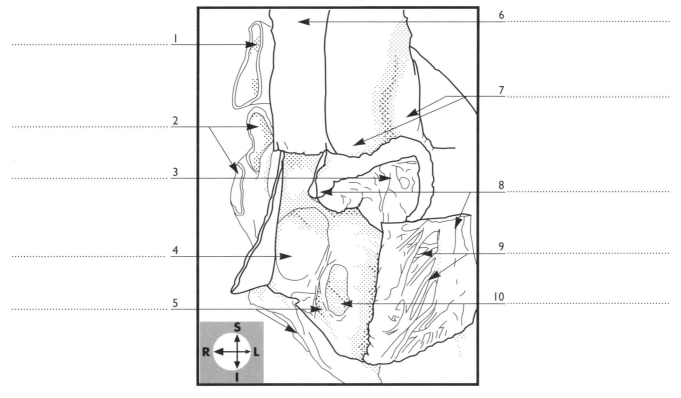

Fig. 2.7 The pulmonary and aortic valves seen from above

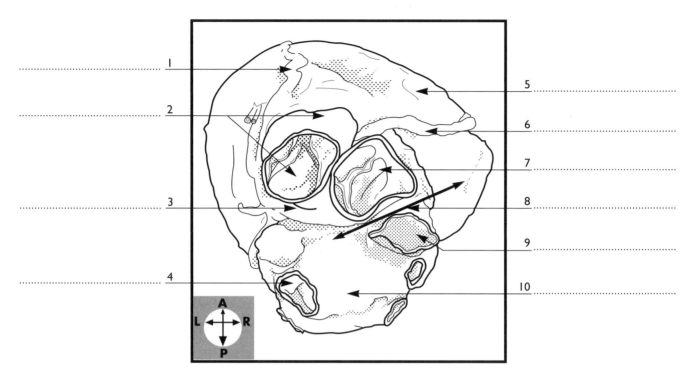

Fig. 2.8 Interior of the left ventricle seen after removal of part of its wall

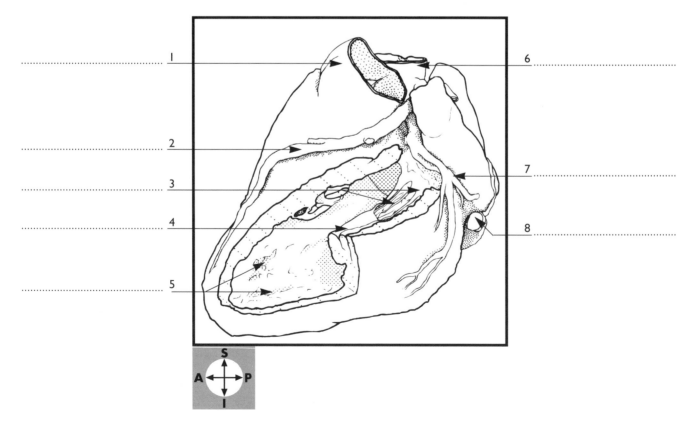

Fig. 2.9 Section through the heart shows the apical portions of the left and right ventricles

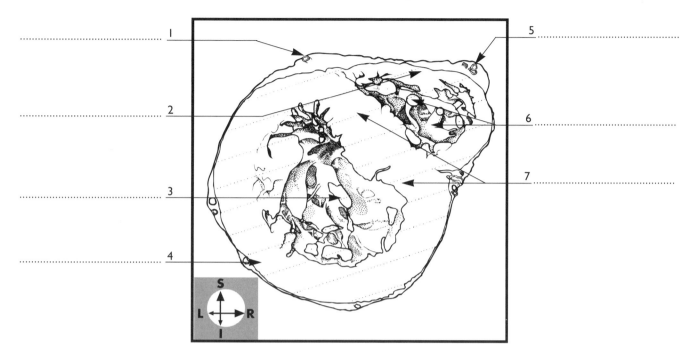

1 ....
2 ....
3 ....
4 ....
5 ....
6 ....
7 ....

Fig. 2.10 Anterior view of the aorta, pulmonary trunk and ligamentum arteriosum

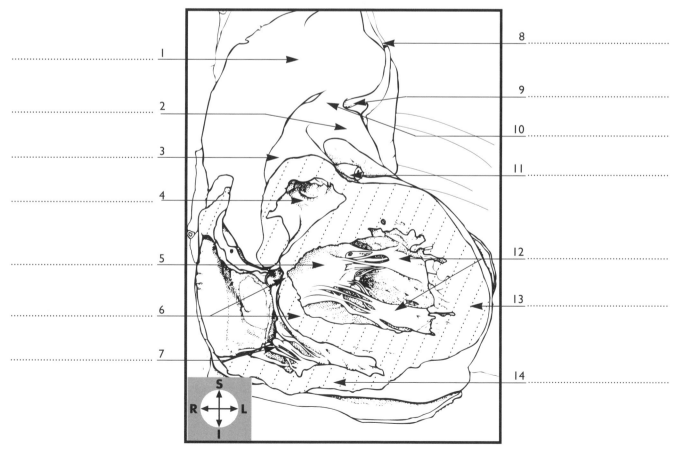

1 ....
2 ....
3 ....
4 ....
5 ....
6 ....
7 ....
8 ....
9 ....
10 ....
11 ....
12 ....
13 ....
14 ....

Fig. 2.11 Right and left coronary arteries and their branches on the anterior surface of the heart

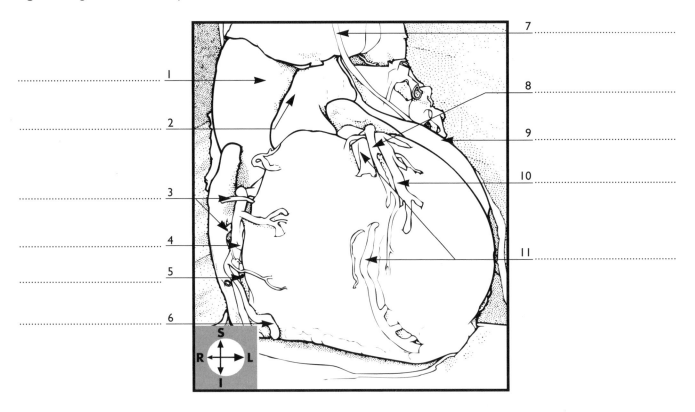

Fig. 2.12 Left coronary artery and its branches viewed from the left

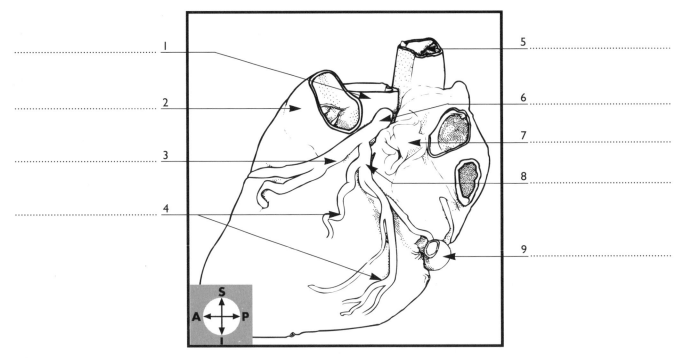

Fig. 2.13 Oblique view of the coronary sinus lying in the atrioventricular groove

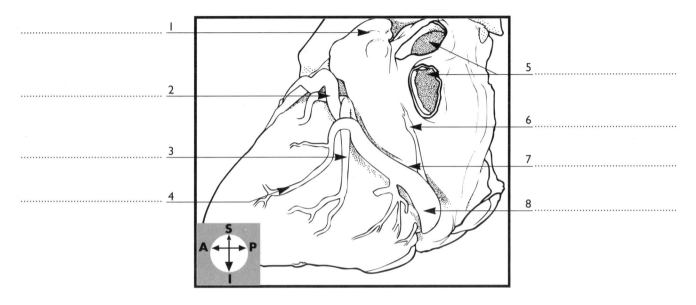

Fig. 2.14 Oblique view of the arch of the aorta showing the courses of the left vagus and phrenic nerves

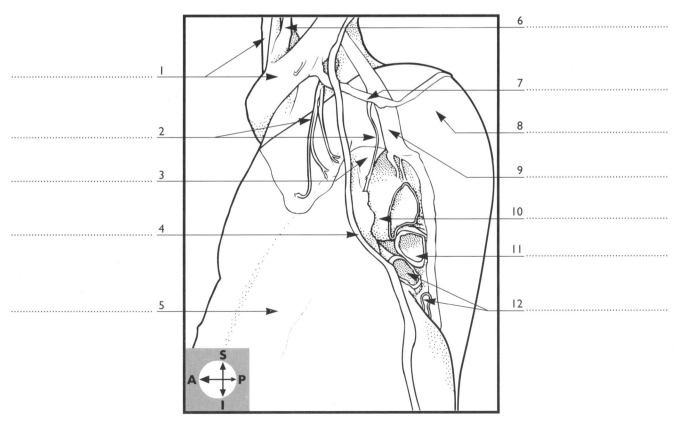

Fig. 2.15 Oblique view of the intrathoracic course of the left phrenic nerve

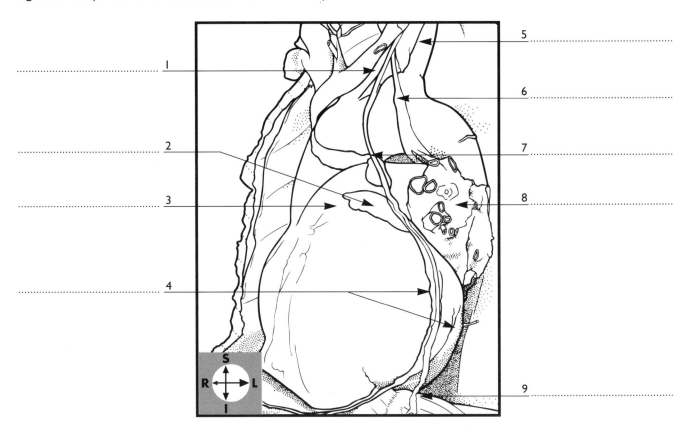

Fig. 2.16 Intrathoracic part of the oesophagus and accompanying vagus nerves after removal of the main bronchi and the lower part of the trachea

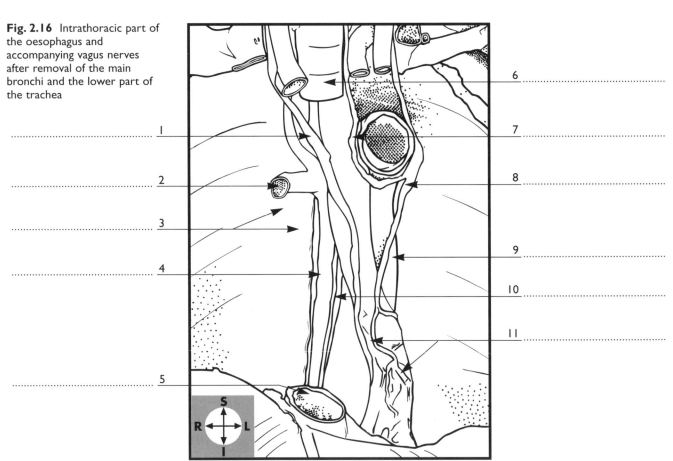

Fig. 2.17 Azygos vein, right intercostal nerves and posterior intercostal vessels exposed after removal of the parietal pleura

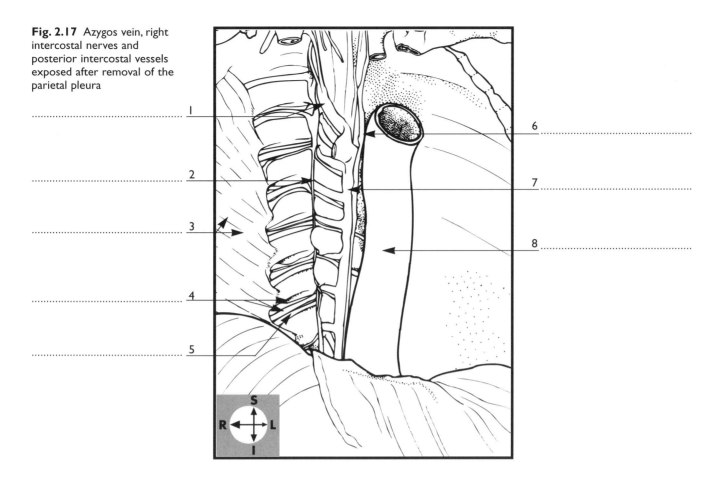

Fig. 2.18 Oblique view of left sympathetic trunk, hemiazygos vein, intercostal nerves and posterior intercostal vessels after removal of the descending aorta and parietal pleura on the left side of the midline

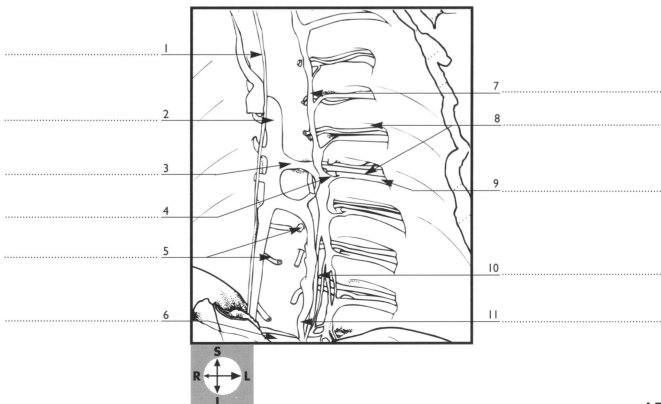

3. Upper Limb

Fig. 3.1 Distribution of cutaneous nerves in the upper limb

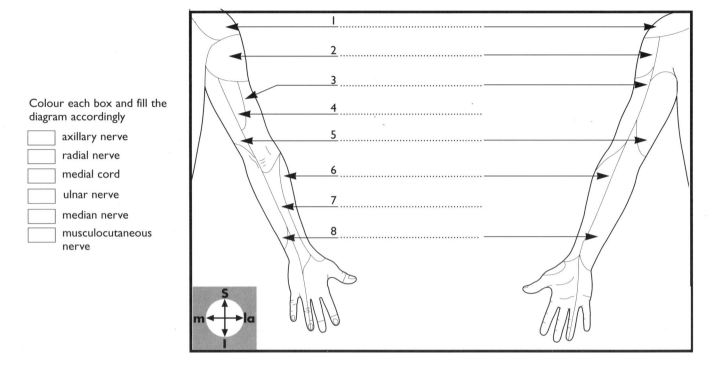

Colour each box and fill the diagram accordingly

- axillary nerve
- radial nerve
- medial cord
- ulnar nerve
- median nerve
- musculocutaneous nerve

Fig. 3.2 Principal arteries of the upper limb. No muscular branches are shown

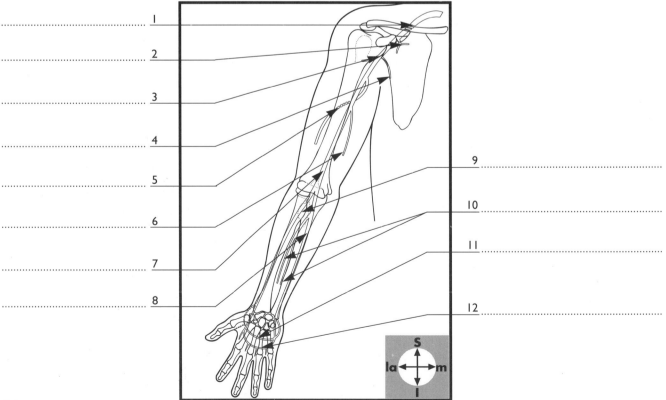

Fig. 3.3 Principal veins of the upper limb

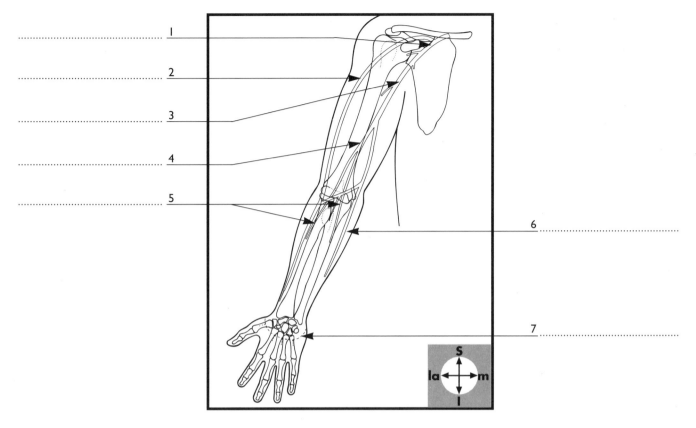

.... 1

.... 2

.... 3

.... 4

.... 5

6 ....

7 ....

Fig. 3.4 Course of the median nerve

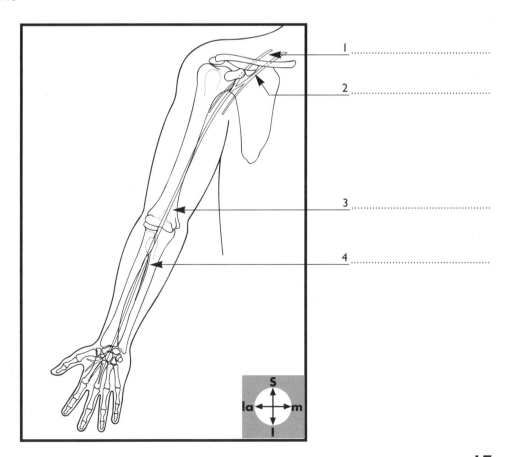

1 ....

2 ....

3 ....

4 ....

Fig. 3.5 Course of the musculocutaneous and ulnar nerves

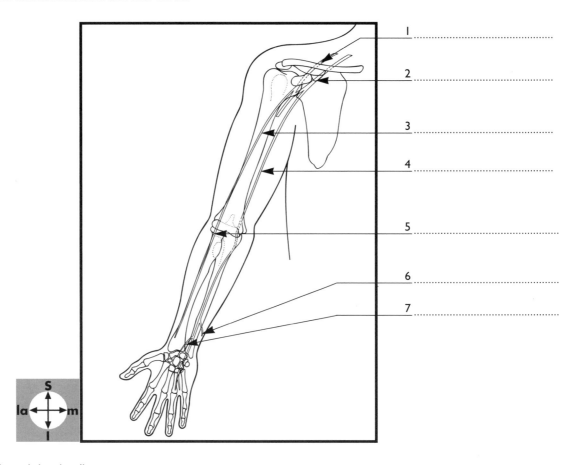

Fig 3.6 Course of the radial and axillary nerves

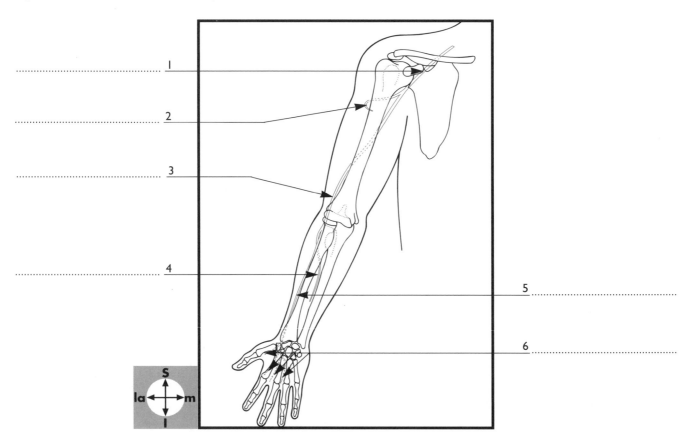

Fig. 3.7 Transverse section through the axilla

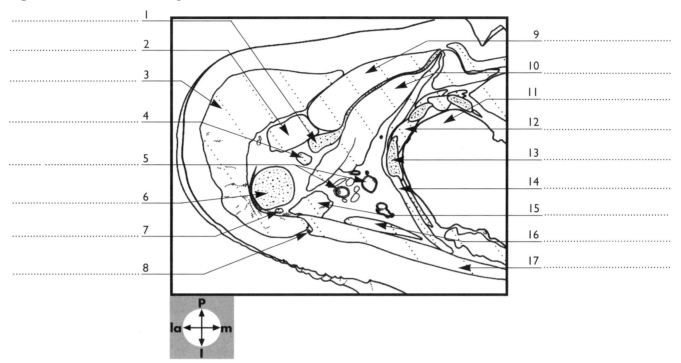

Fig. 3.8 Some posterior branches of the brachial plexus after removal of the more anterior parts of the plexus

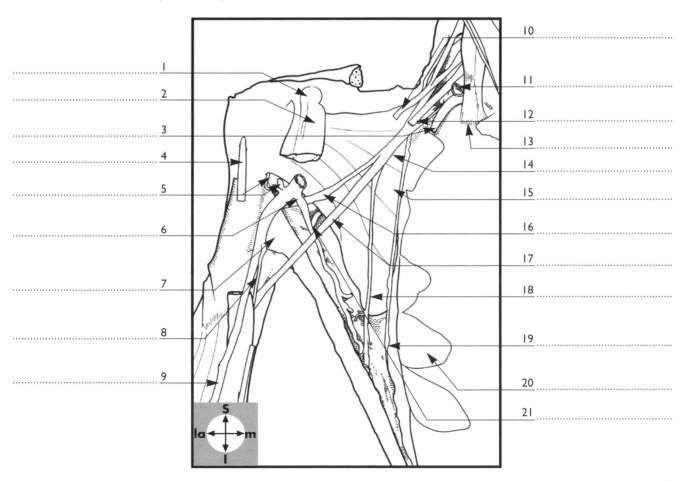

Fig. 3.9 Components of the brachial plexus

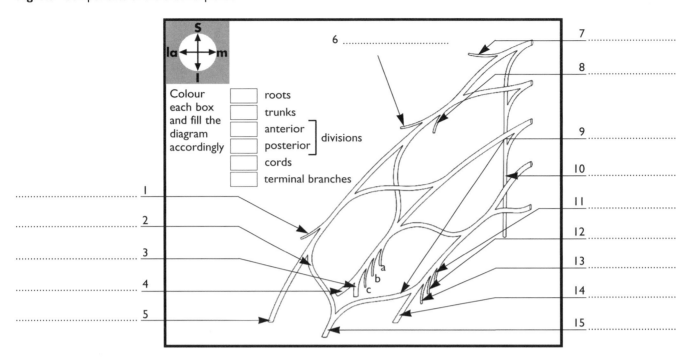

Colour each box and fill the diagram accordingly

☐ roots
☐ trunks
☐ anterior ⎫
☐ posterior ⎬ divisions
☐ cords
☐ terminal branches

Fig. 3.10 Anterior view of biceps after removal of deep fascia and anterior fibres of deltoid

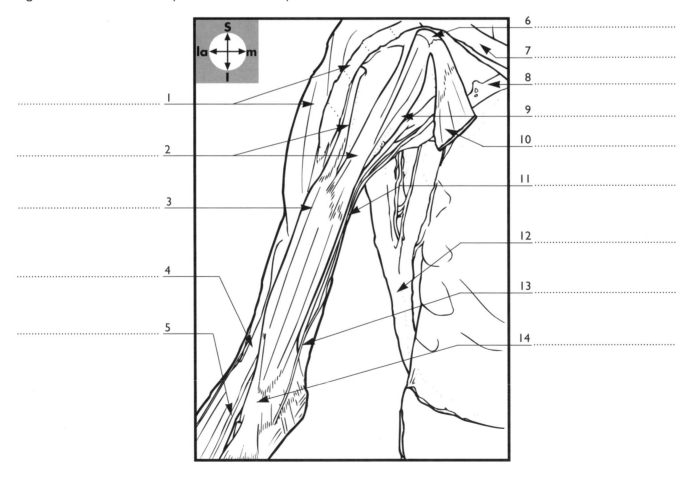

Fig. 3.11 The cubital fossa. The aponeurosis of biceps and deep fascia have been removed

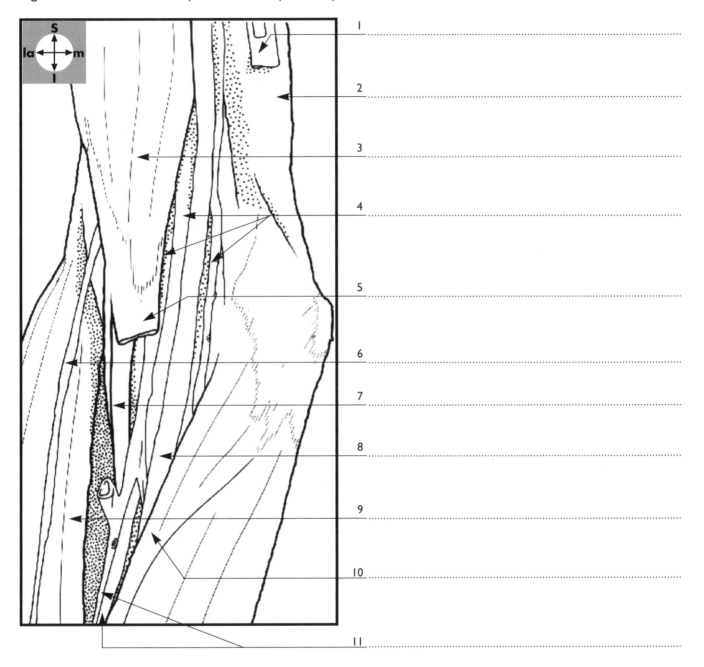

1 ....

2 ....

3 ....

4 ....

5 ....

6 ....

7 ....

8 ....

9 ....

10 ....

11 ....

Fig. 3.12 Flexor digitorum profundus and flexor pollicis longus exposed by removal of the superficial flexors

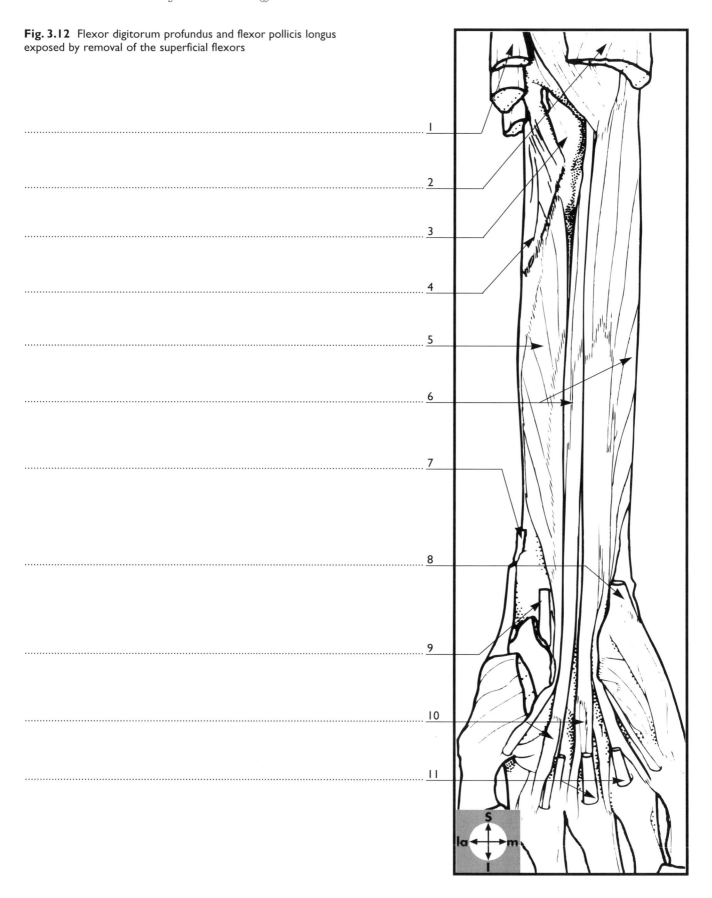

1 ....

2 ....

3 ....

4 ....

5 ....

6 ....

7 ....

8 ....

9 ....

10 ....

11 ....

Fig. 3.13 Anterior aspects of radius, ulna and distal end of humerus showing areas of muscle attachment

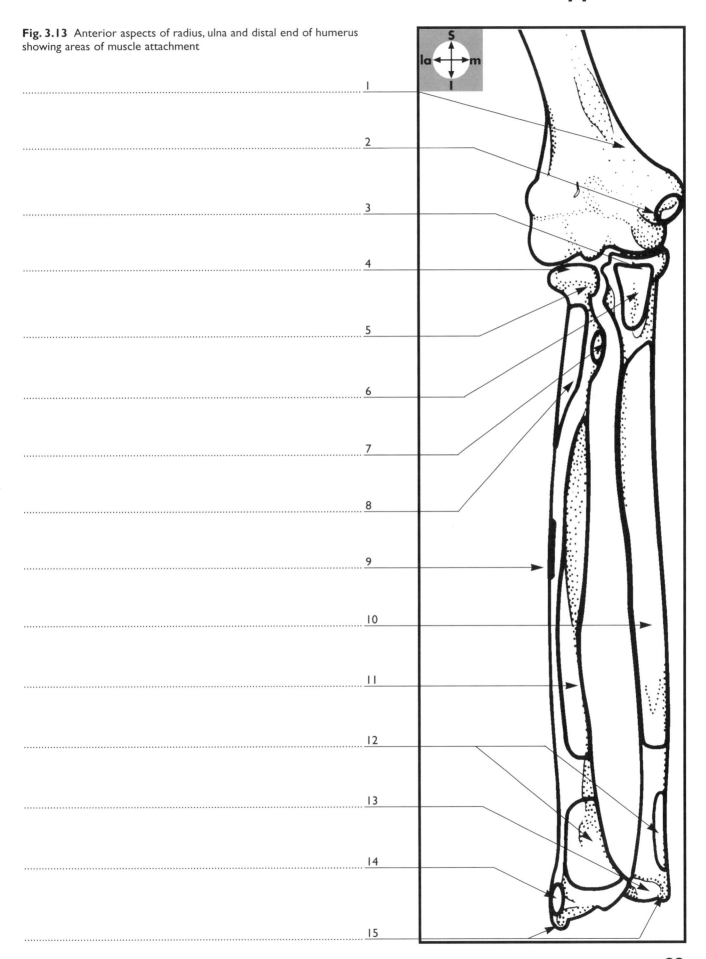

1 ....

2 ....

3 ....

4 ....

5 ....

6 ....

7 ....

8 ....

9 ....

10 ....

11 ....

12 ....

13 ....

14 ....

15 ....

Fig. 3.14 Vessels and nerves of the anterior compartment of the forearm. Most venae comitantes have been removed

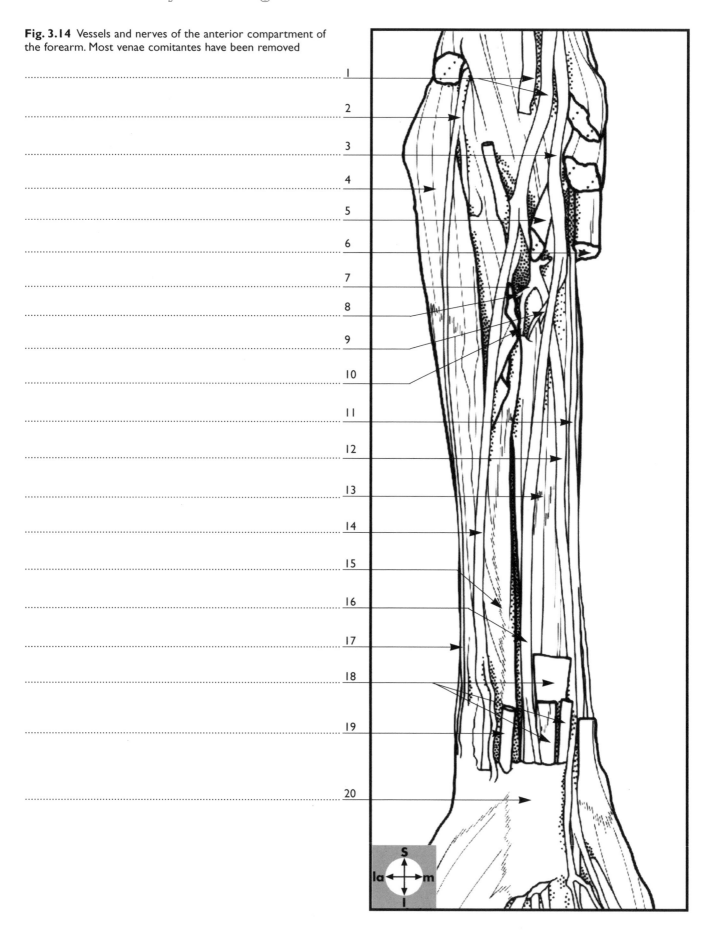

1 ....

2 ....

3 ....

4 ....

5 ....

6 ....

7 ....

8 ....

9 ....

10 ....

11 ....

12 ....

13 ....

14 ....

15 ....

16 ....

17 ....

18 ....

19 ....

20 ....

Fig. 3.15 Palmar aponeurosis exposed by removal of skin and superficial fascia

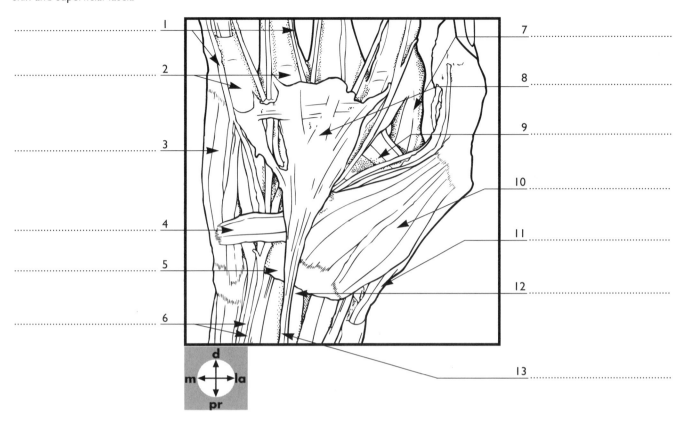

Fig. 3.16 Transverse section through the index finger at the level of the proximal phalanx

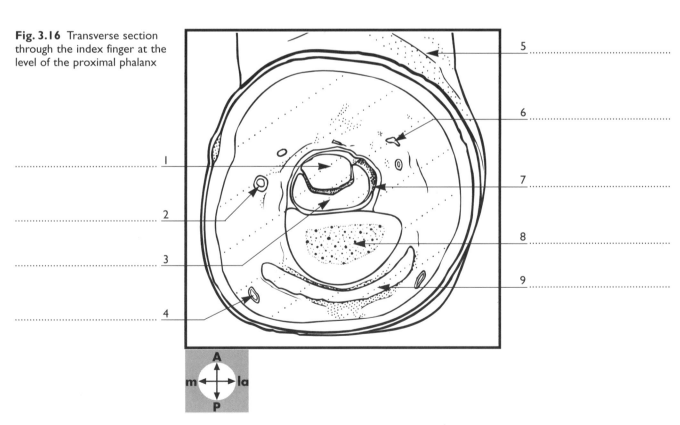

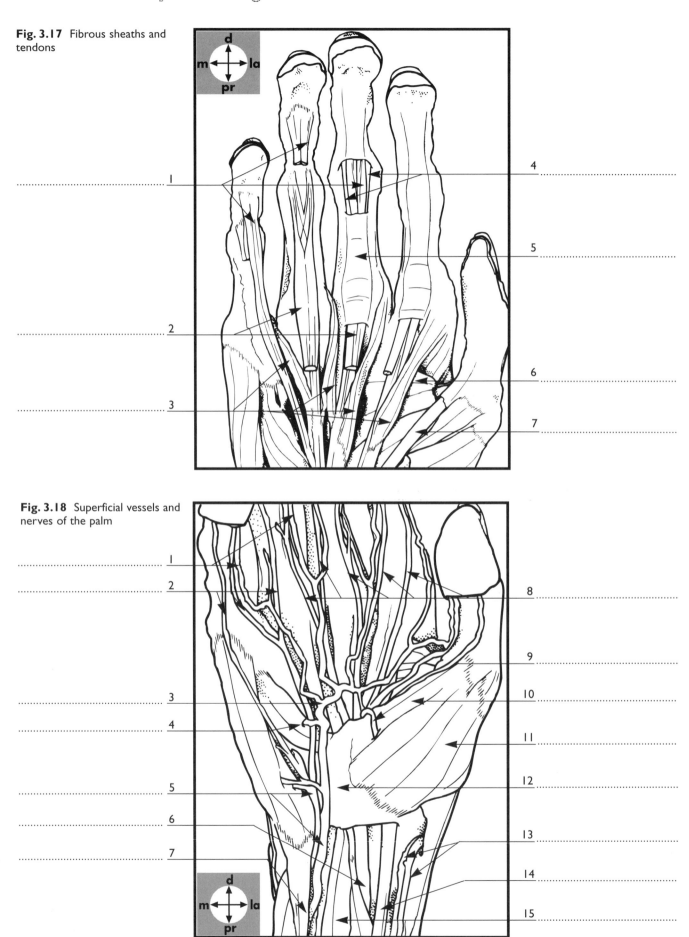

Fig. 3.17 Fibrous sheaths and tendons

Fig. 3.18 Superficial vessels and nerves of the palm

Fig. 3.19 Deep dissection of the palm

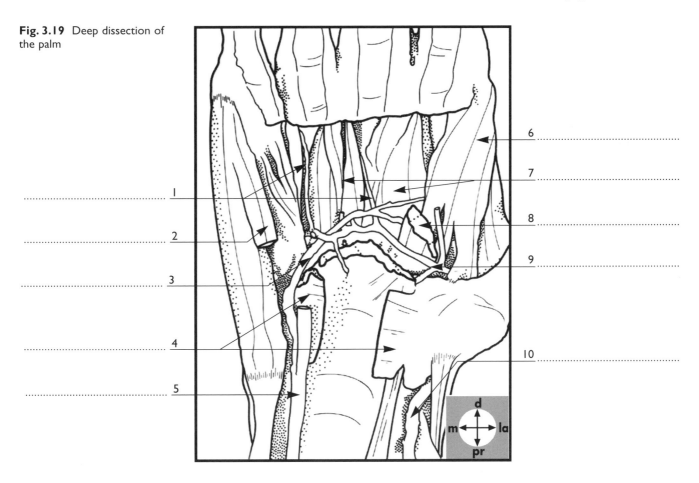

Fig. 3.20 Superficial back muscles

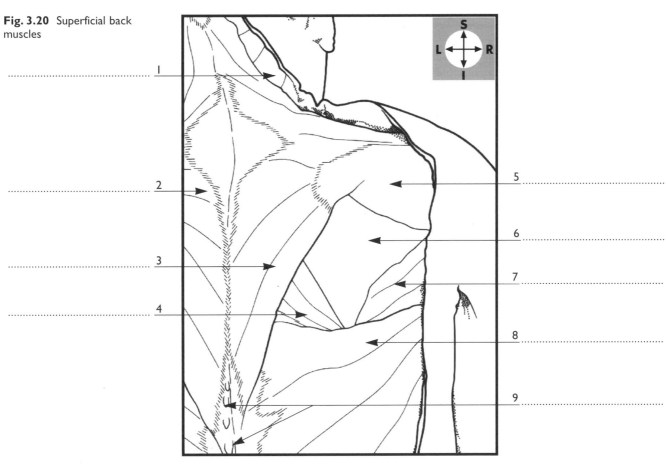

Fig. 3.21 Anterior view of subscapularis

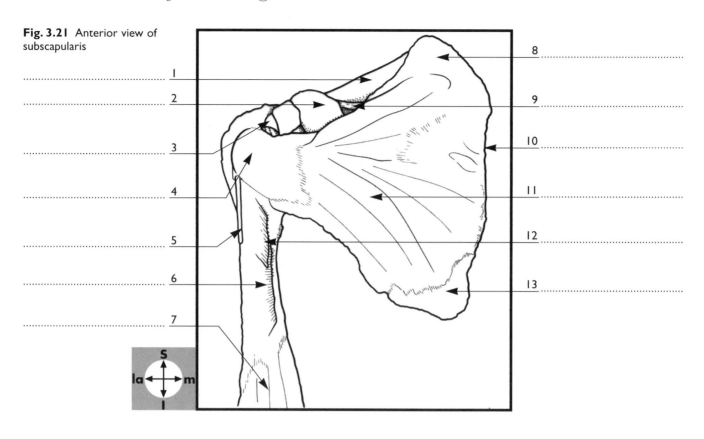

Fig. 3.22 Teres major and minor and the intermuscular spaces

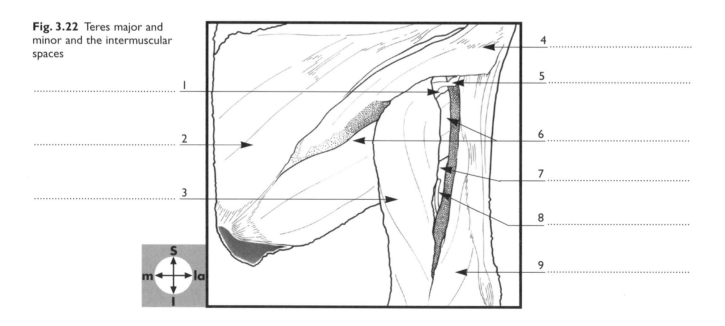

Fig. 3.23 Superficial muscles of the posterior compartment exposed by removal of deep fascia and the extensor retinaculum

....

....

....

....

....

....

....

....

....

....

....

....

....

....

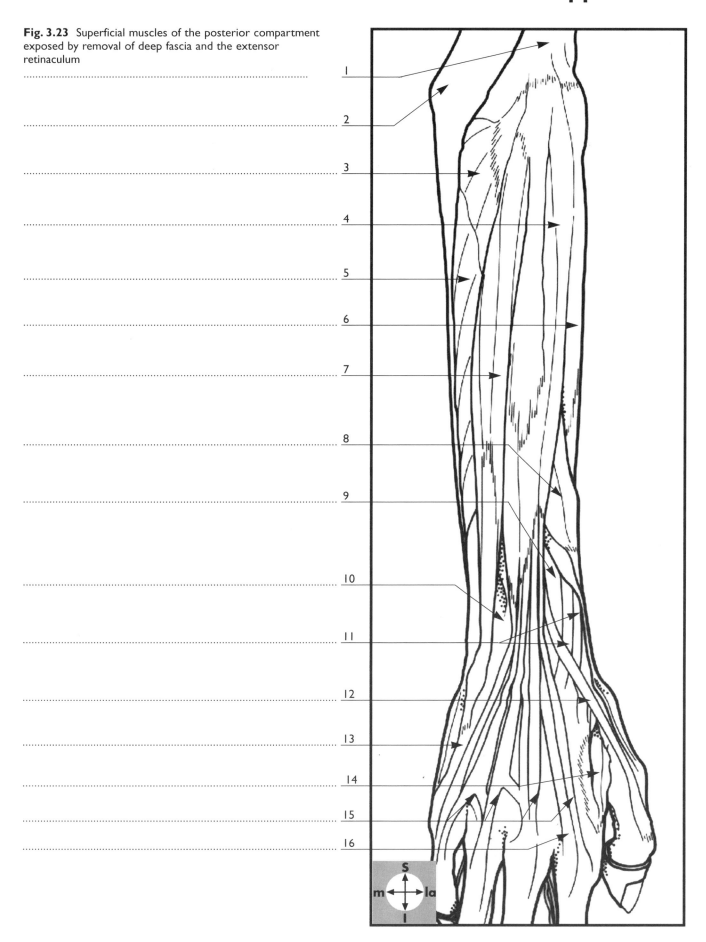

Fig. 3.24 Anterior aspect of the forearm

.... 1

.... 2

.... 3

.... 4

.... 5

.... 6

.... 7

.... 8

.... 9

.... 10

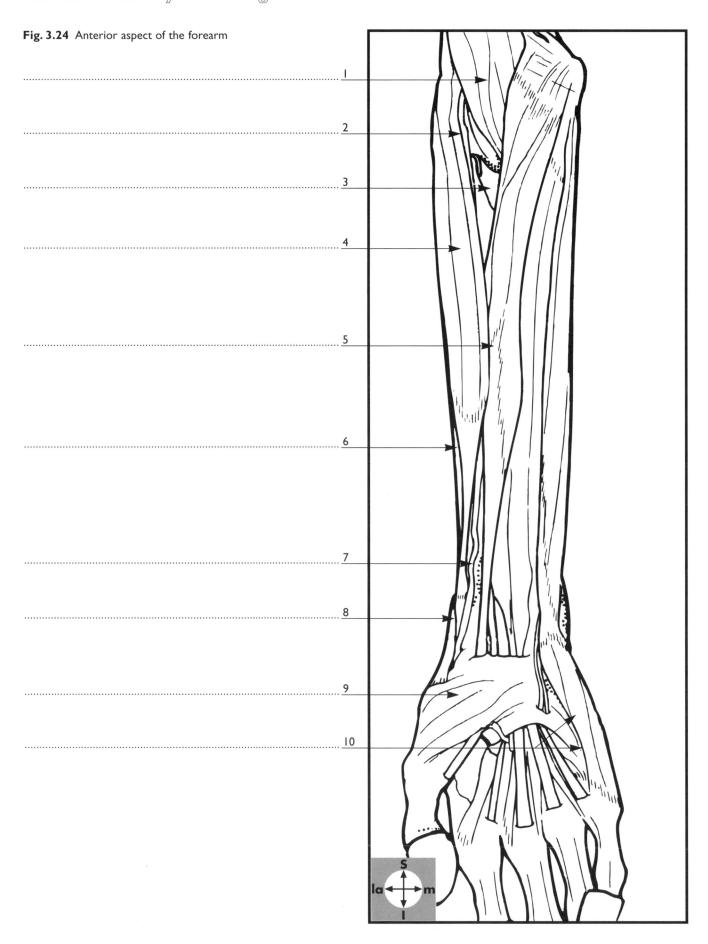

Fig. 3.25 Muscles and tendons on the lateral aspect of the forearm

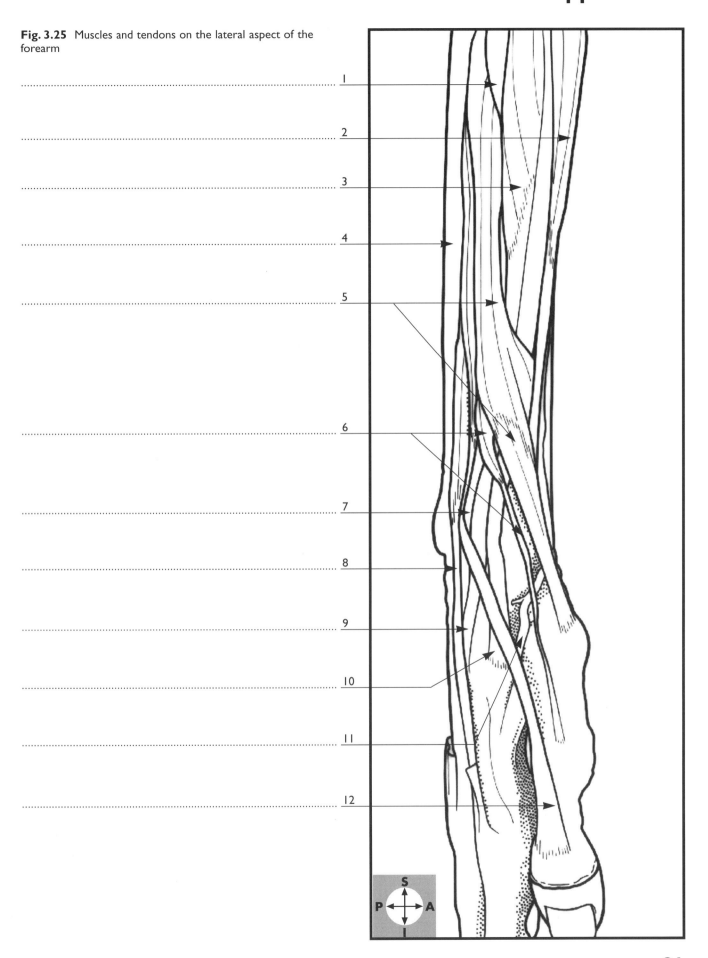

1 ....

2 ....

3 ....

4 ....

5 ....

6 ....

7 ....

8 ....

9 ....

10 ....

11 ....

12 ....

Fig. 3.26 Extensor retinaculum and extensor tendons exposed by removal of superficial fascia

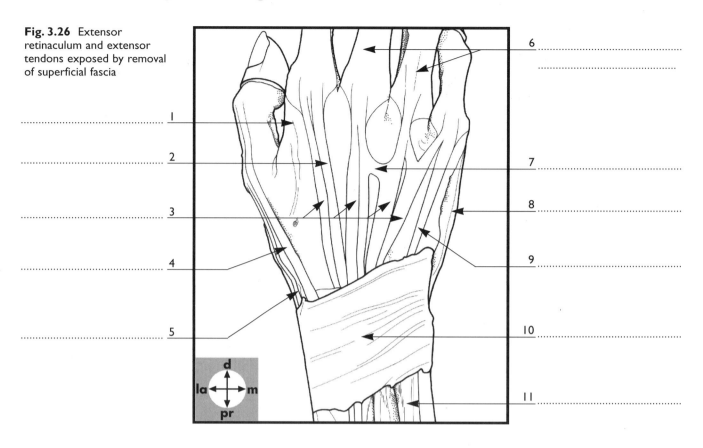

1
2
3
4
5
6
7
8
9
10
11

d
la — m
pr

Fig. 3.27 Transverse section at the level of the humeral head showing the relations of the shoulder joint

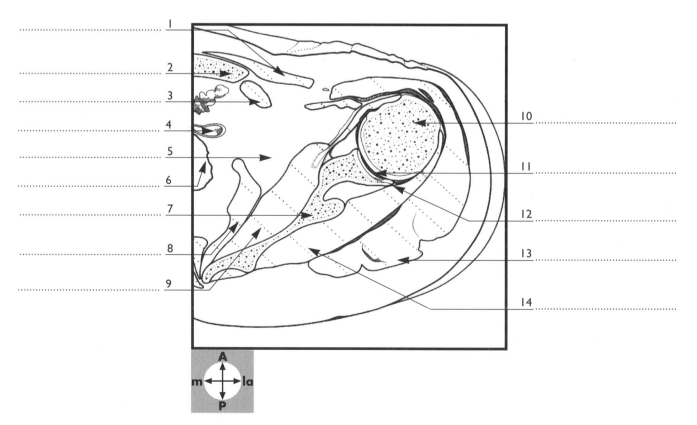

1
2
3
4
5
6
7
8
9
10
11
12
13
14

A
m — la
P

Fig. 3.28 Posterior aspect of the shoulder joint. The acromion and parts of the rotator cuff muscles have been excised

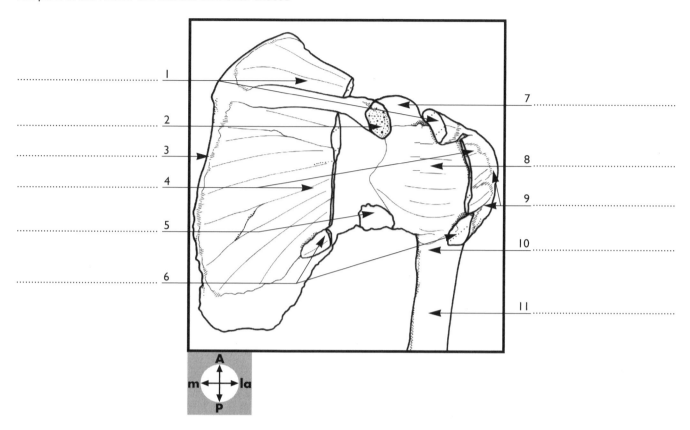

Fig. 3.29 Oblique longitudinal section of elbow (extended) and proximal radioulnar joints showing the articular surfaces and relations of the joints

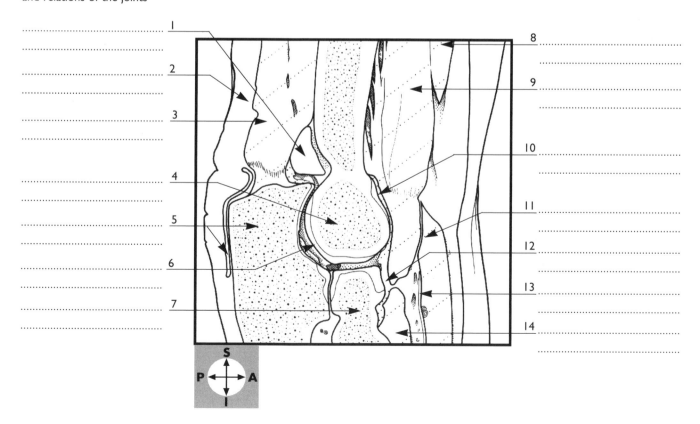

Fig. 3.30 Transverse section through the carpus showing the carpal tunnel and its contents

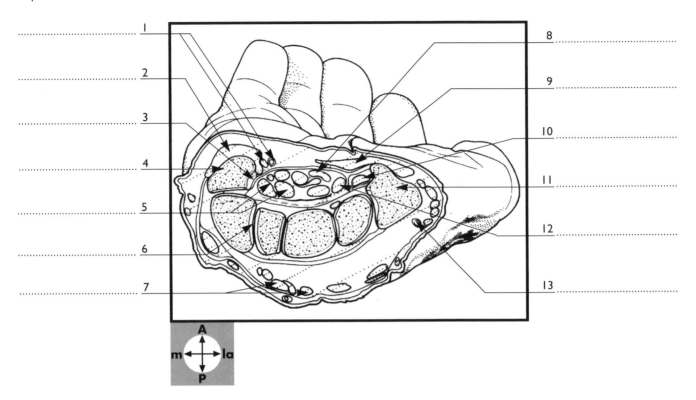

Fig. 3.31 Flexor retinaculum and the superficial relations and structures entering the carpal tunnel

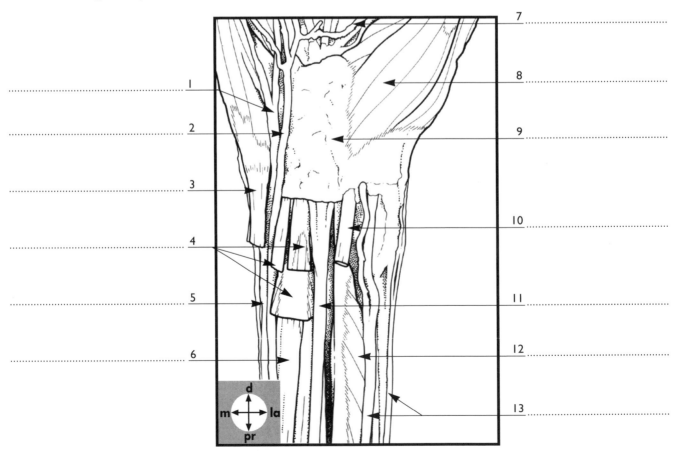

4. Abdomen

Fig. 4.1 The digestive organs within the abdomen

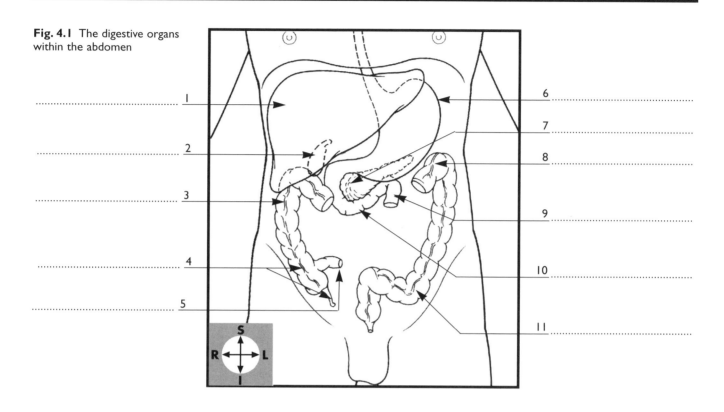

1 ....

2 ....

3 ....

4 ....

5 ....

6 ....

7 ....

8 ....

9 ....

10 ....

11 ....

Fig. 4.2 The kidneys and related organs

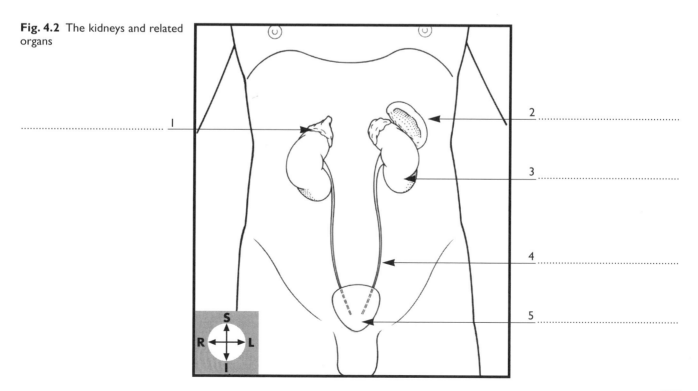

1 ....

2 ....

3 ....

4 ....

5 ....

Fig. 4.3 Principal arteries of the abdomen

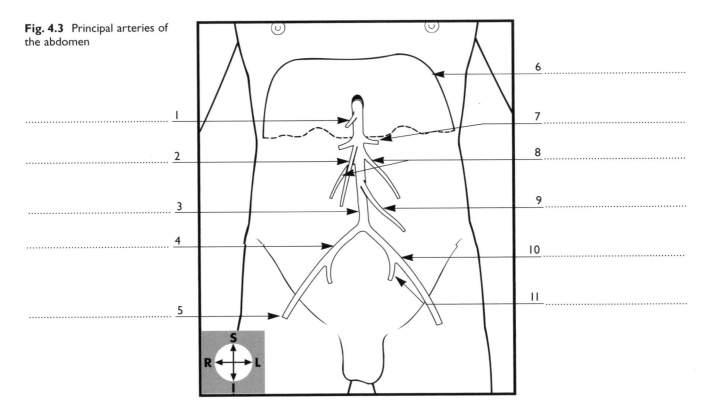

Fig. 4.4 Principal systemic veins of the abdomen

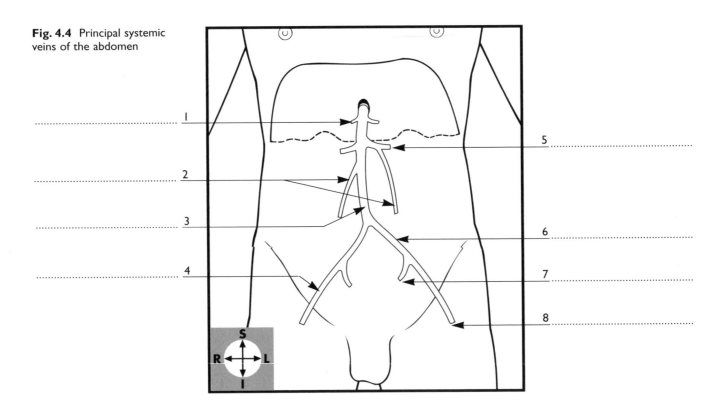

Fig. 4.5 The portal venous system

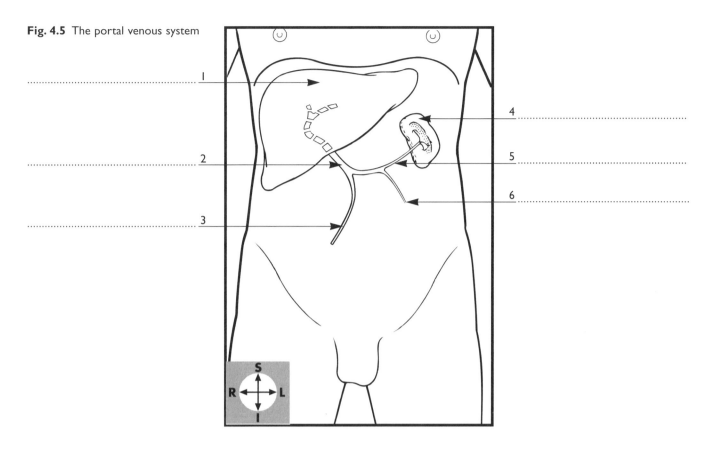

Fig. 4.6 Rectus abdominis muscles and neurovascular plane

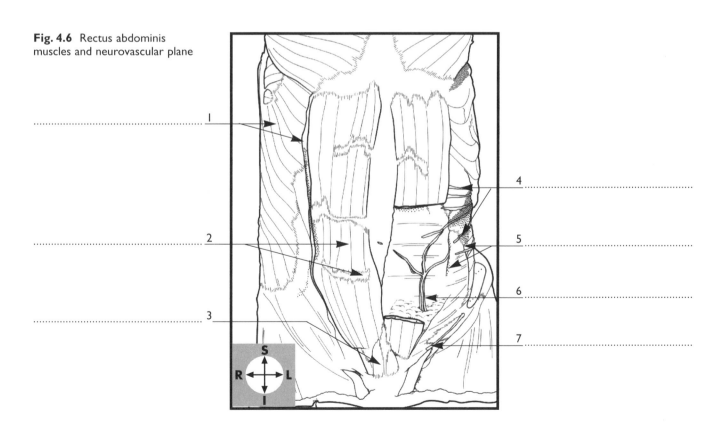

Fig. 4.7 Position of the inguinal canal and its superficial and deep rings in relation to the inguinal ligaments, the pubis and the iliac crest

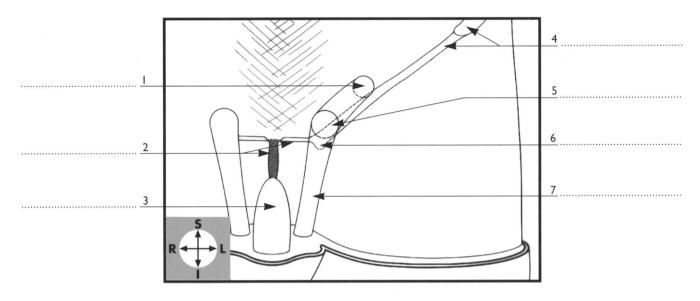

Fig. 4.8 Lower fibres of internal oblique and part of the spermatic cord have been excised to reveal the posterior wall and floor of the inguinal canal

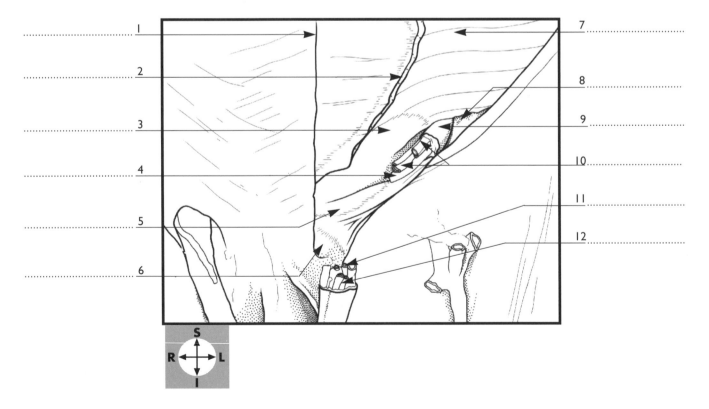

Fig. 4.9 Transverse section through the scrotum

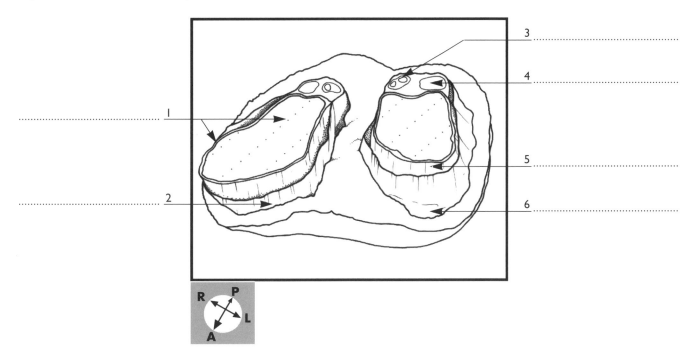

Fig. 4.10 Transverse section through the abdomen at the level of the second lumbar vertebra

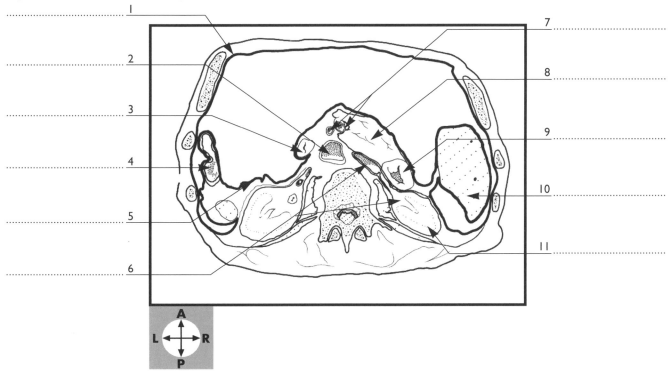

Fig. 4.11 Transverse section at the level of the disc between the twelfth thoracic and first lumbar vertebrae

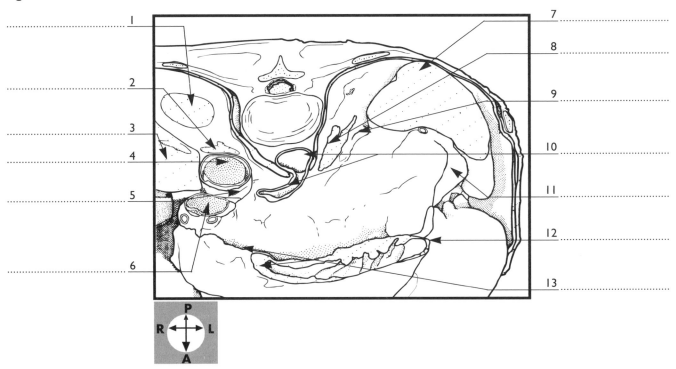

Fig. 4.12 The stomach and some of its relations

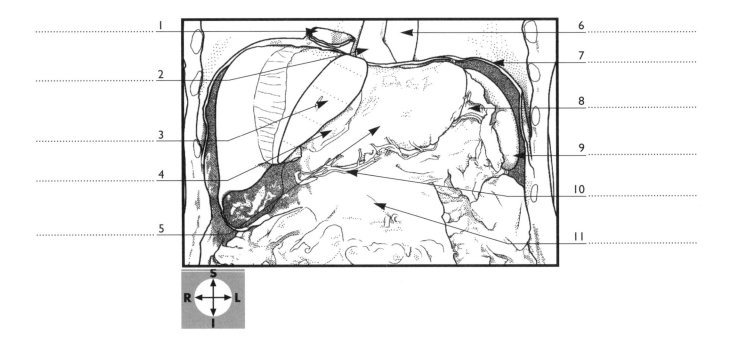

Fig. 4.13 The spleen and its vessels and their relationship to the diaphragm, pancreas and left kidney

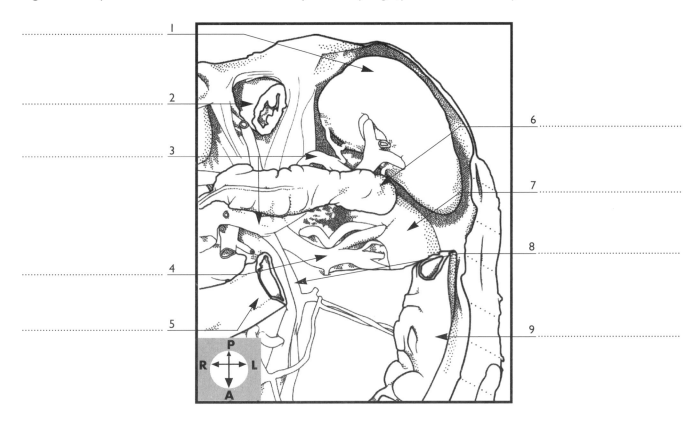

Fig. 4.14 Principal relations and parts of the pancreas

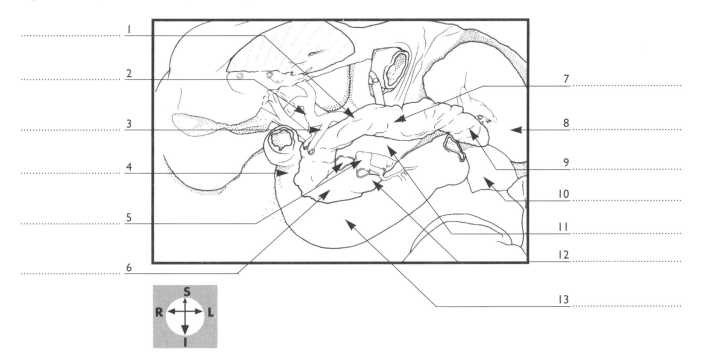

Fig. 4.15 Inferior view of liver and gall bladder showing porta hepatis and visceral surface

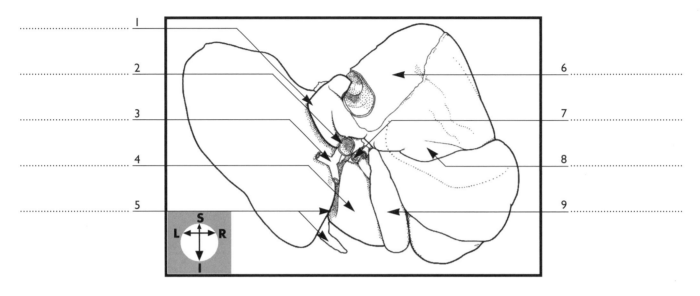

Fig. 4.16 Posterior view of liver, stomach and lesser omentum

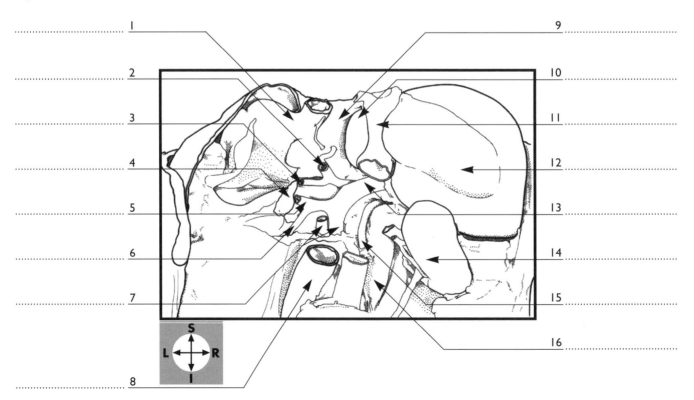

Fig. 4.17 Course and branches of the hepatic artery

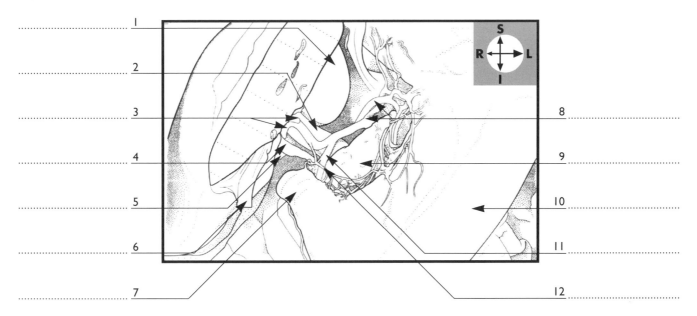

Fig. 4.18 Jejunum and ileum

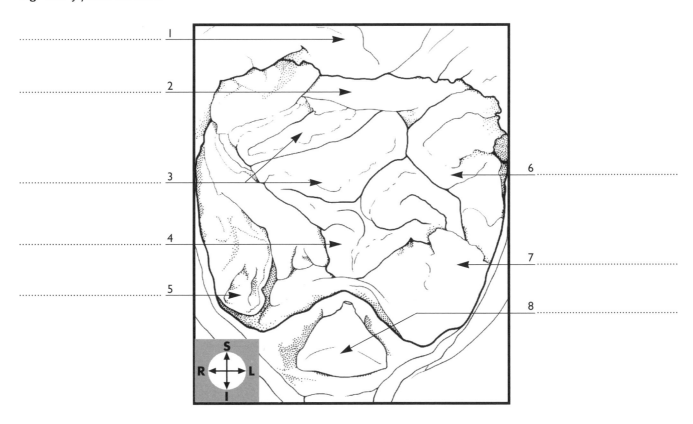

Fig. 4.19 Superior mesenteric artery and its branches

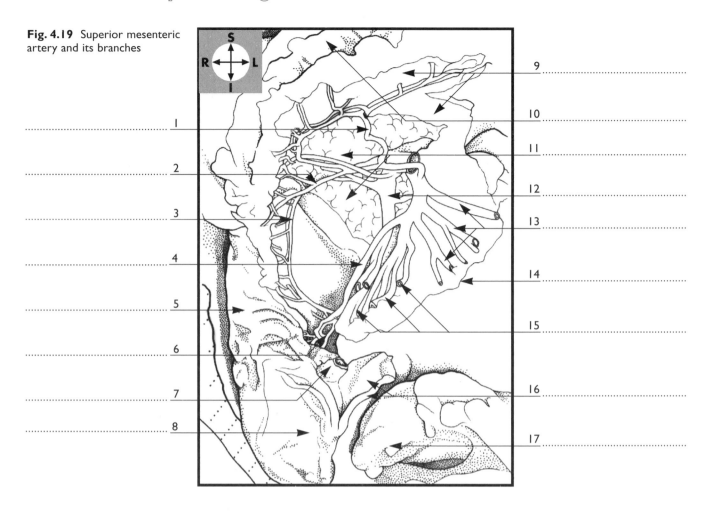

Fig. 4.20 Blood supply to the left colic flexure, descending colon and sigmoid colon

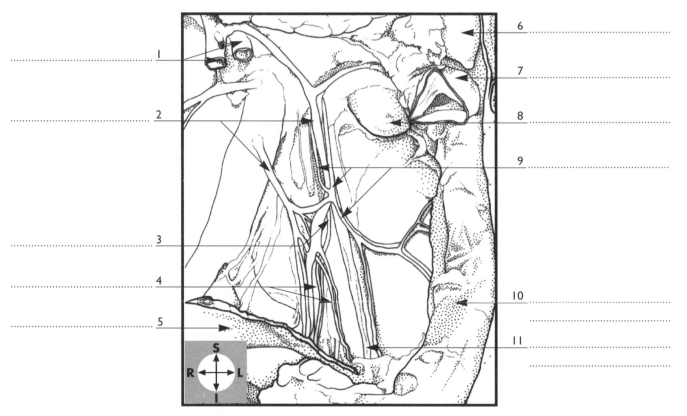

Fig. 4.21 The portal and splenic veins

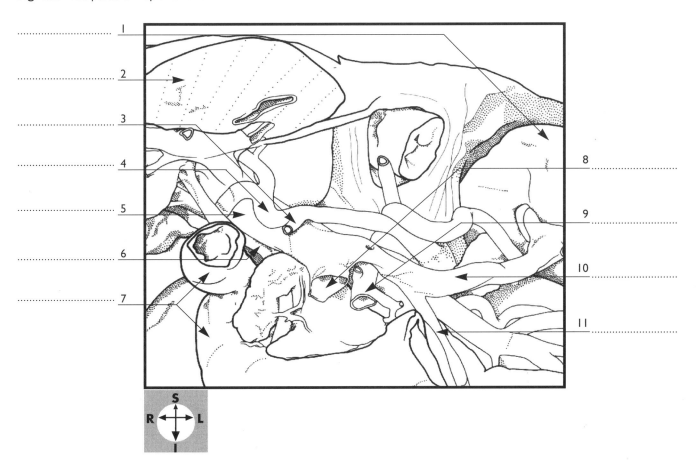

Fig. 4.22 The kidneys and suprarenal glands and some of the vessels associated with them

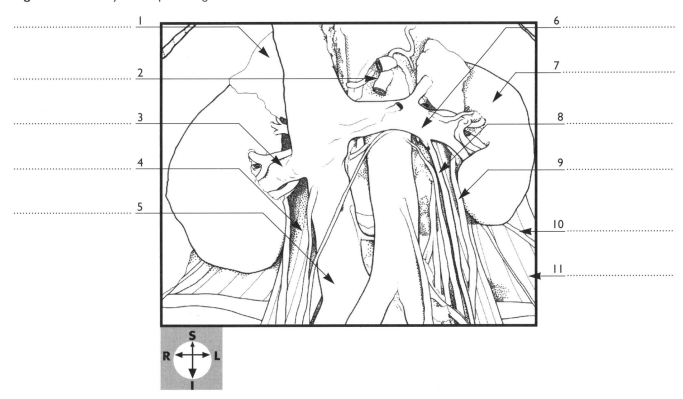

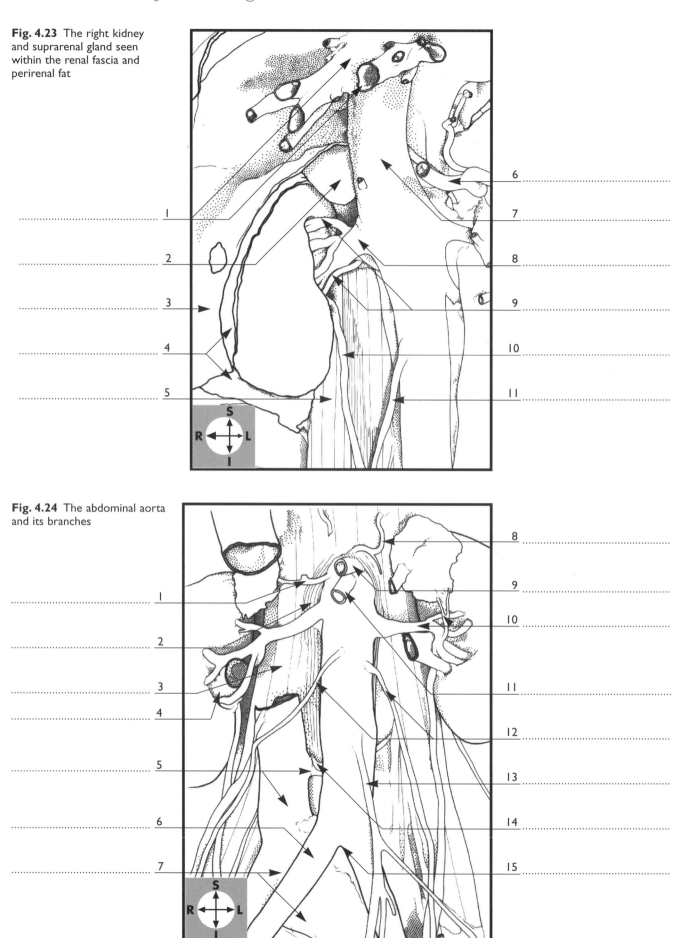

Fig. 4.23 The right kidney and suprarenal gland seen within the renal fascia and perirenal fat

1
2
3
4
5
6
7
8
9
10
11

Fig. 4.24 The abdominal aorta and its branches

1
2
3
4
5
6
7
8
9
10
11
12
13
14
15

Fig. 4.25 Lymphatic vessels and nodes lying on the right side of the aorta

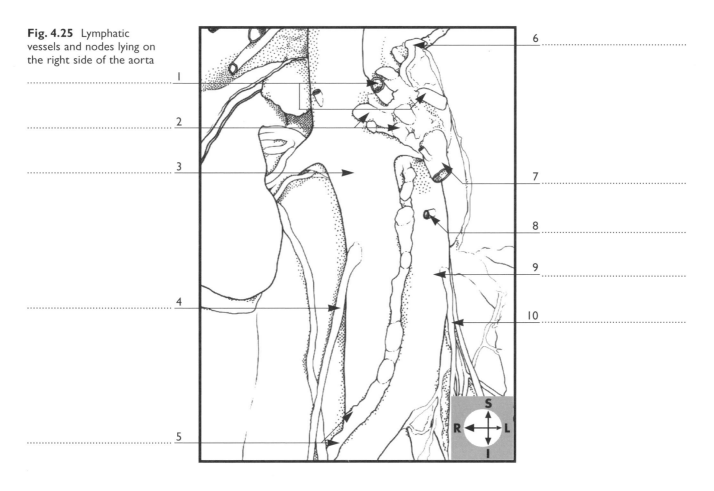

1
2
3
4
5
6
7
8
9
10

Fig. 4.26 The muscles and nerves of the posterior abdominal wall

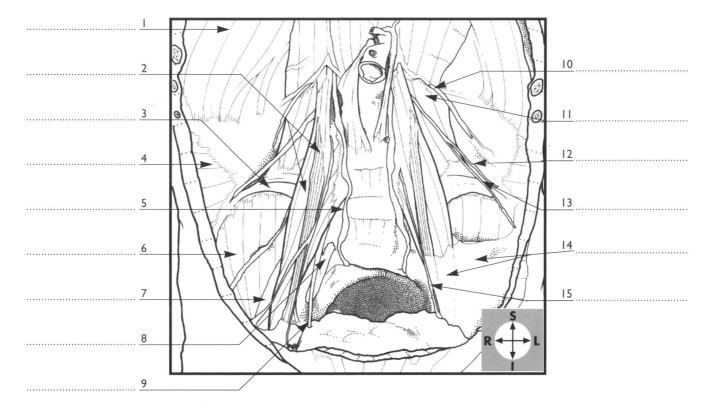

1
2
3
4
5
6
7
8
9
10
11
12
13
14
15

Fig. 4.27 The lumbar plexus

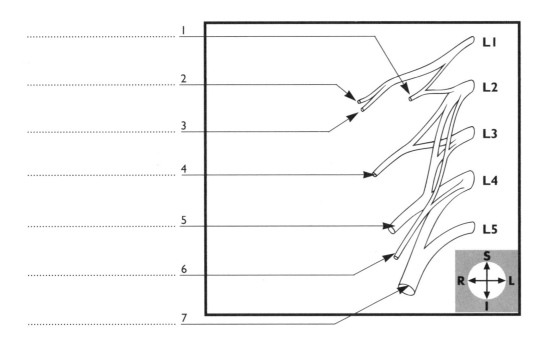

Fig. 4.28 Abdominal surface of the diaphragm after removal of the peritoneum

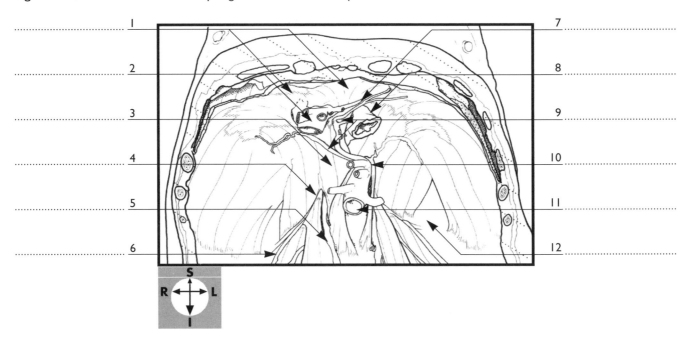

5. Pelvis & Perineum

Fig. 5.1 The internal iliac artery and some of its branches to the pelvis, perineum and lower limb

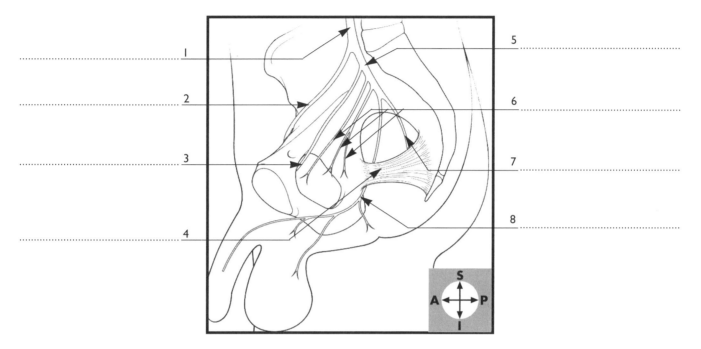

Fig. 5.2 Superior view of the peritoneum and organs within the female pelvis

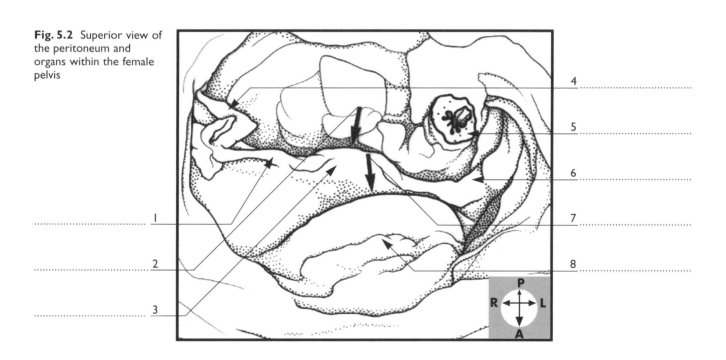

Fig. 5.3 The uterus and vagina in sagittal section

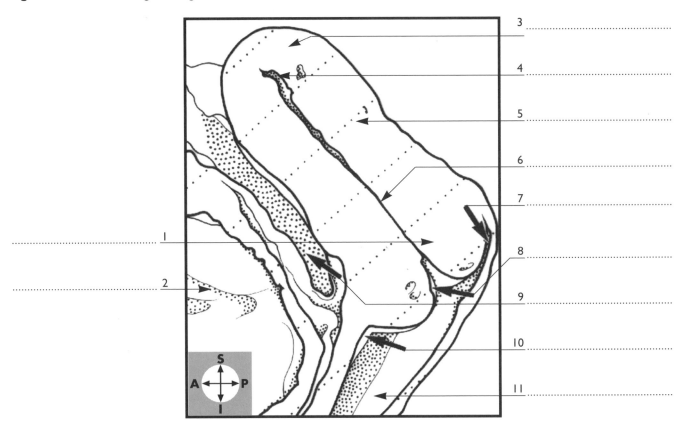

Fig. 5.4 Pelvic blood vessels in the female

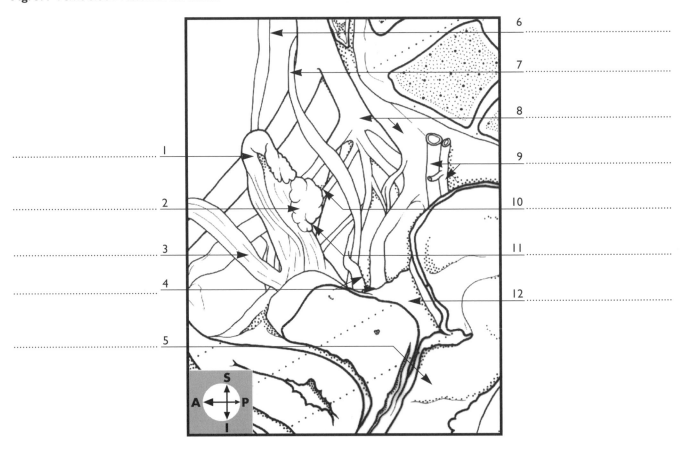

Fig. 5.5 The female urethra and its relationship to the vagina and the levator ani muscles

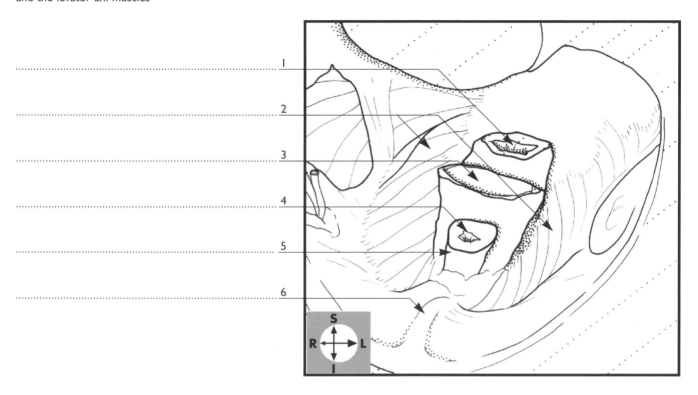

Fig. 5.6 The male urethra in sagittal section

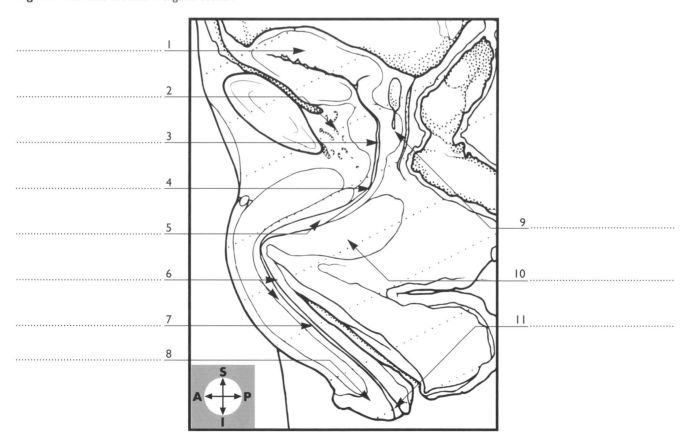

Fig. 5.7 The bladder, prostate, seminal vesicles and vasa deferentia

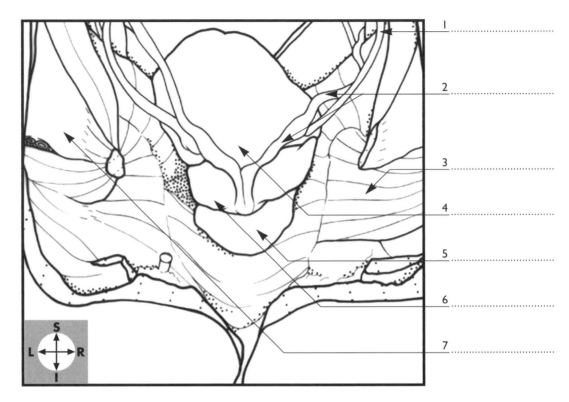

1 ....

2 ....

3 ....

4 ....

5 ....

6 ....

7 ....

Fig. 5.8 Structures on lateral wall of male pelvis

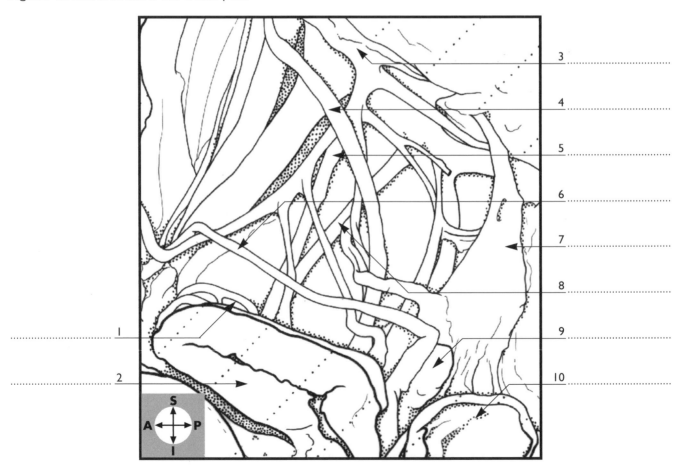

3 ....

4 ....

5 ....

6 ....

7 ....

8 ....

9 ....

10 ....

.... 1

.... 2

Fig. 5.9 Coronal section through the anal canal and ischiorectal fossae

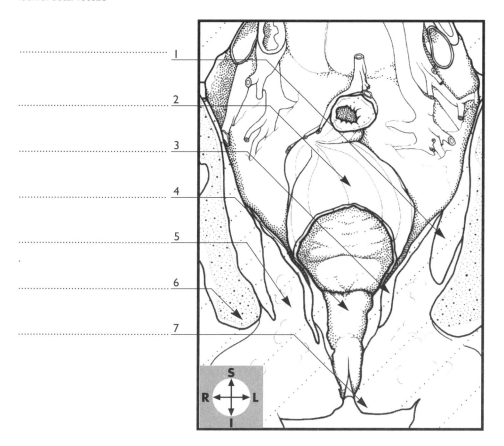

Fig. 5.10 Root of the penis

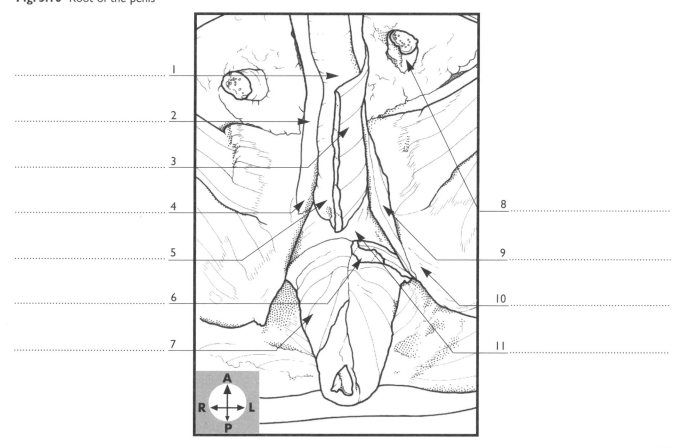

Fig. 5.11 Deep dissection of the female perineum. The glans, shaft and left crus of the clitoris have been exposed

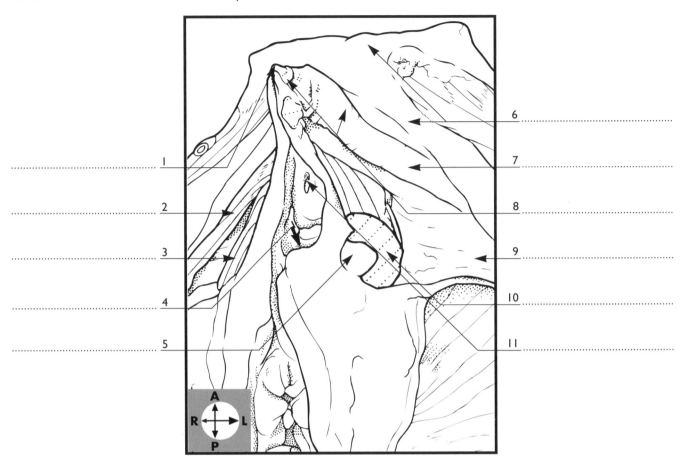

1 ....

2 ....

3 ....

4 ....

5 ....

6 ....

7 ....

8 ....

9 ....

10 ....

11 ....

6. Lower Limb

Fig. 6.1 The skeleton of the lower limb

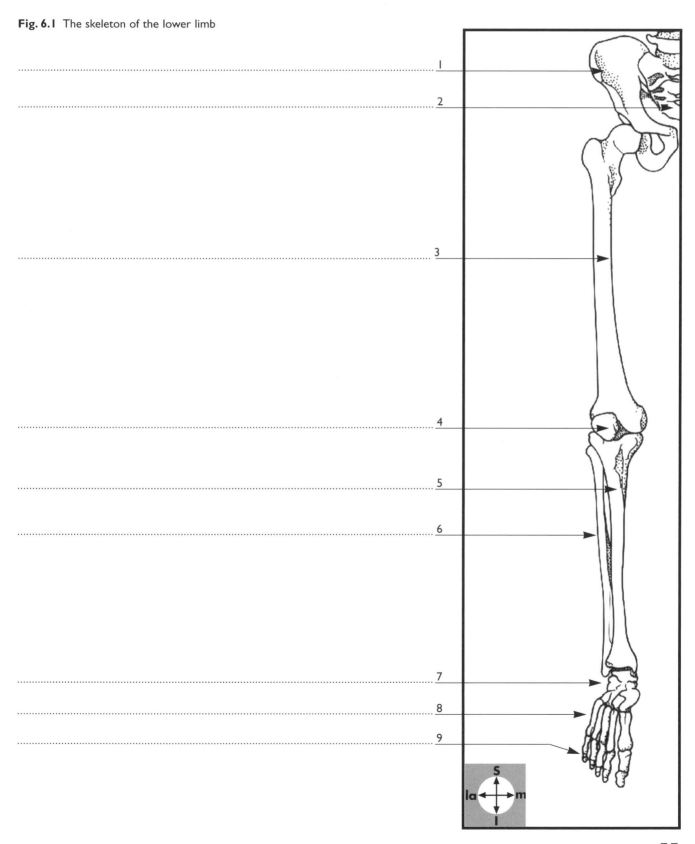

.... 1

.... 2

.... 3

.... 4

.... 5

.... 6

.... 7

.... 8

.... 9

Fig. 6.2 Principal arteries of the lower limb

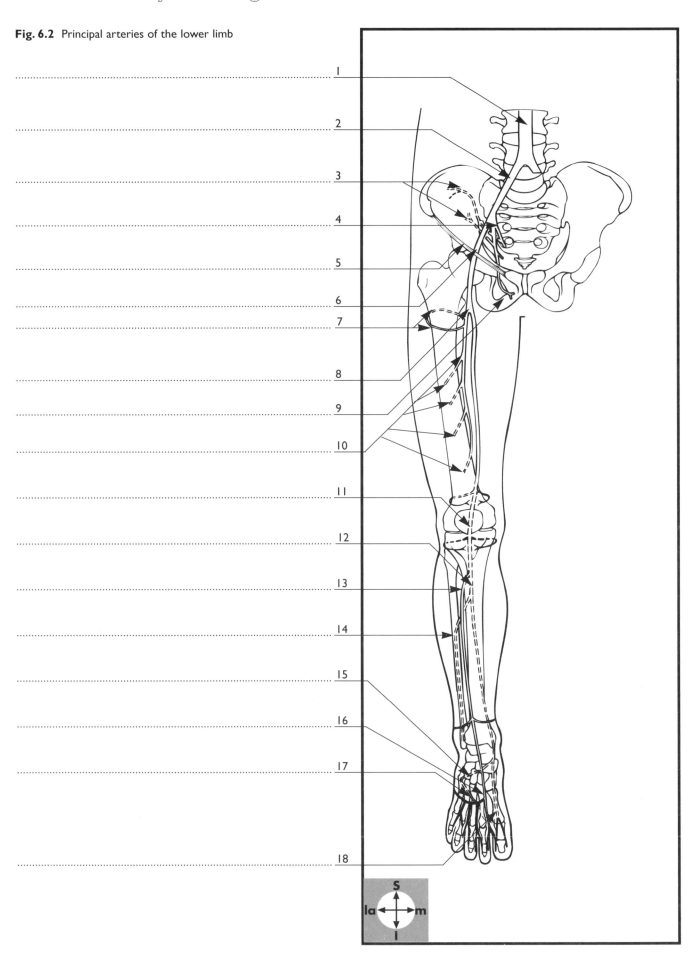

1

2

3

4

5

6

7

8

9

10

11

12

13

14

15

16

17

18

S

la ← → m

I

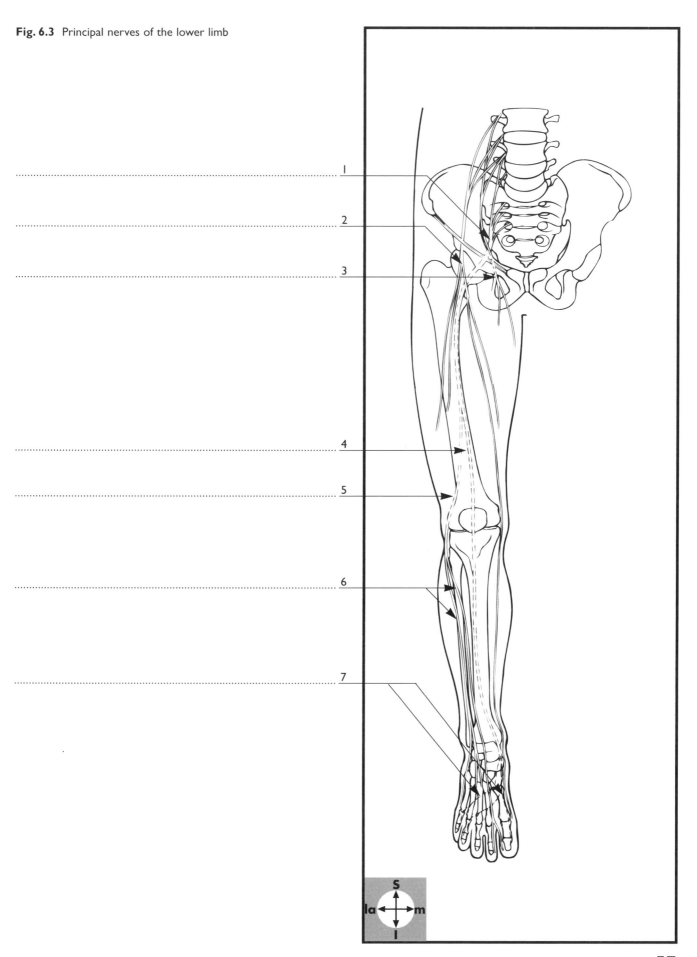

Fig. 6.3 Principal nerves of the lower limb

1 ....

2 ....

3 ....

4 ....

5 ....

6 ....

7 ....

S

la ⟷ m

I

Fig. 6.4 Muscles of the anterior and medial compartments of the thigh

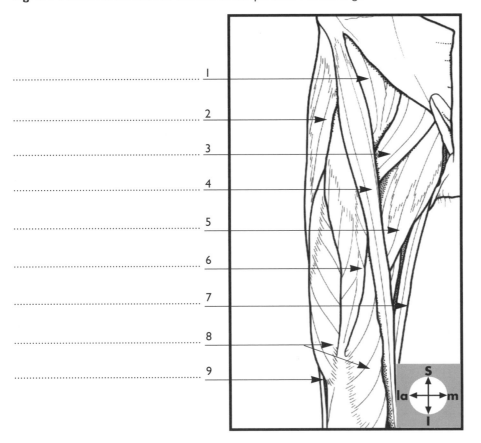

1 ....
2 ....
3 ....
4 ....
5 ....
6 ....
7 ....
8 ....
9 ....

Fig. 6.5 Structures in the femoral triangle and subsartorial canal

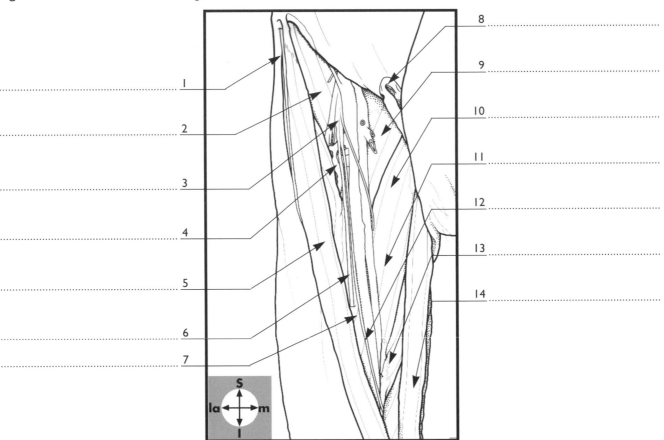

1 ....
2 ....
3 ....
4 ....
5 ....
6 ....
7 ....

8 ....
9 ....
10 ....
11 ....
12 ....
13 ....
14 ....

Fig. 6.6 Divisions of the obturator nerve revealed by removal of the adductor longus and part of the pectineus

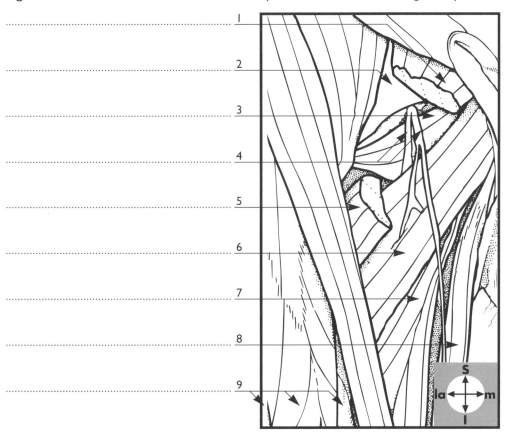

Fig. 6.7 Deep dissection of medial compartment of the thigh showing access of obturator nerve

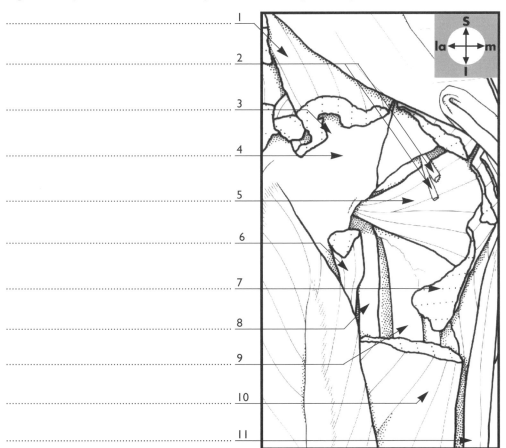

Fig. 6.8 Principal structures in gluteal region beneath gluteus maximus

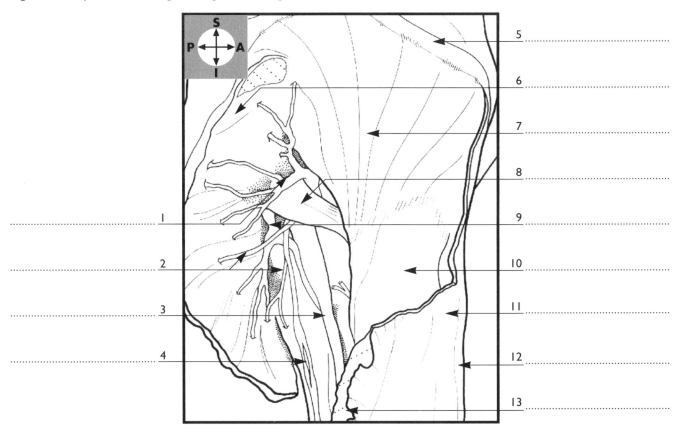

Fig. 6.9 Course of the sciatic nerve through the gluteal region

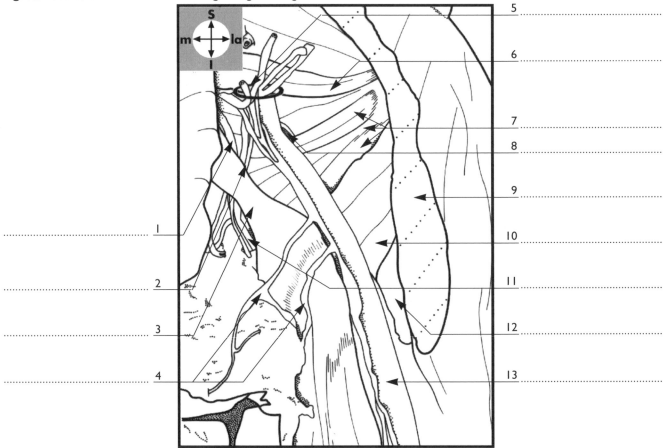

Fig. 6.10 Principal contents of posterior compartment of the thigh

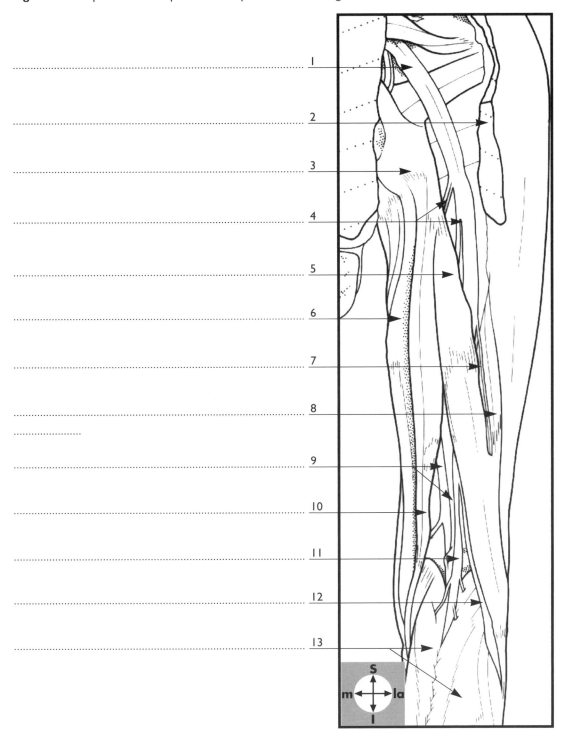

.... 1

.... 2

.... 3

.... 4

.... 5

.... 6

.... 7

....
.... 8

.... 9

.... 10

.... 11

.... 12

.... 13

Fig. 6.11 Principal boundaries and contents of the popliteal fossa

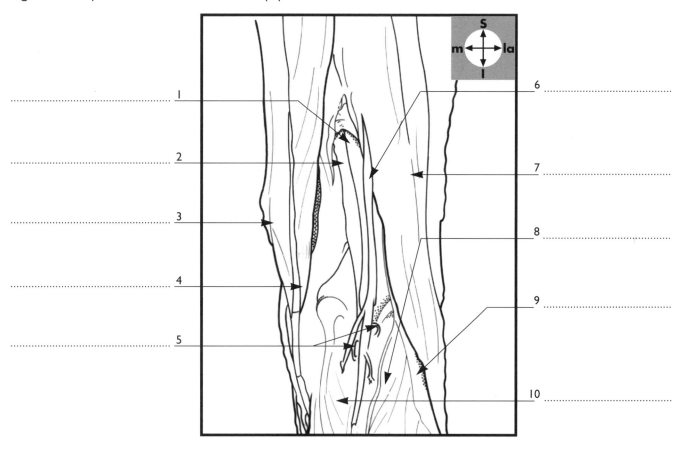

Fig. 6.12 Access of principal nerves and vessels into the posterior compartment of the leg from the popliteal fossa

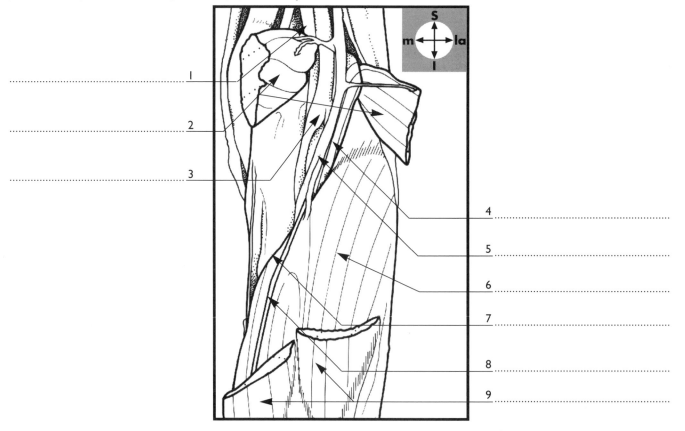

Fig. 6.13 Principal blood vessels and nerves and deeper muscles of the posterior leg compartment

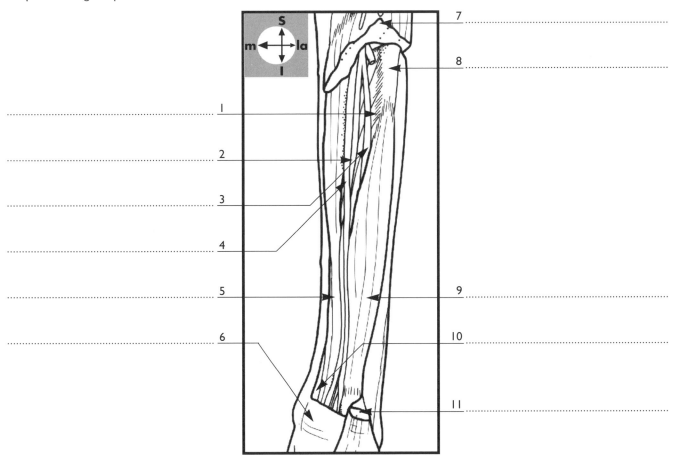

Fig. 6.14 Principal blood vessels, nerves and tendons passing from the posterior leg compartment into the foot

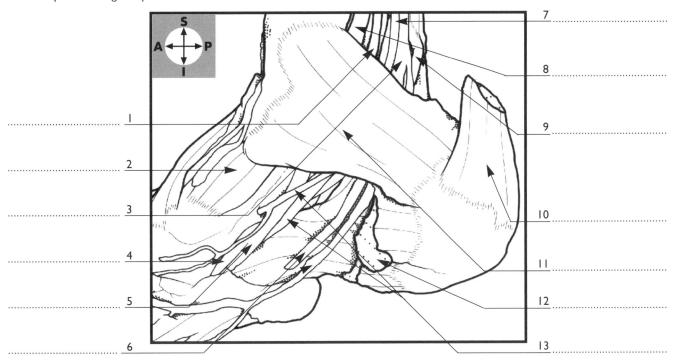

Fig. 6.15 Superficial muscles, tendons and nerves in the sole of the foot

Fig. 6.16 Deeper muscles, tendons and arteries in the sole of the foot

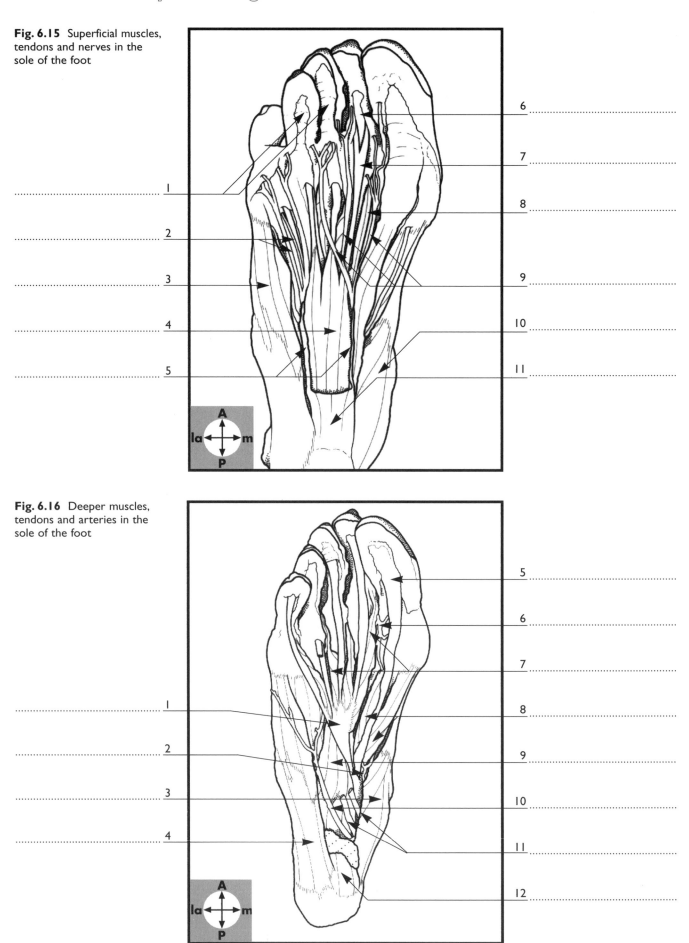

Fig. 6.17 Deep muscles and arteries in the sole of the foot

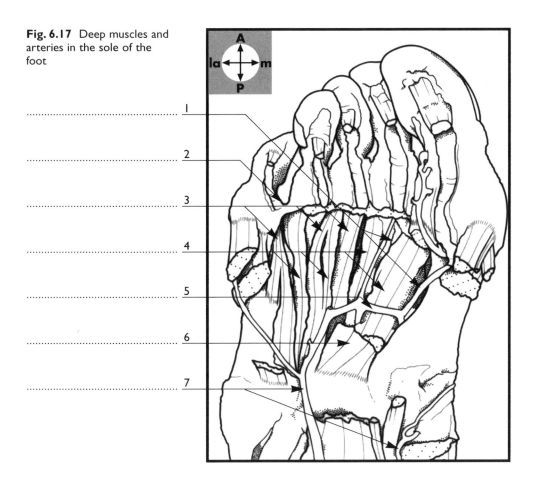

1 ....

2 ....

3 ....

4 ....

5 ....

6 ....

7 ....

Fig. 6.18 Deepest tendons and ligaments in the sole of the foot

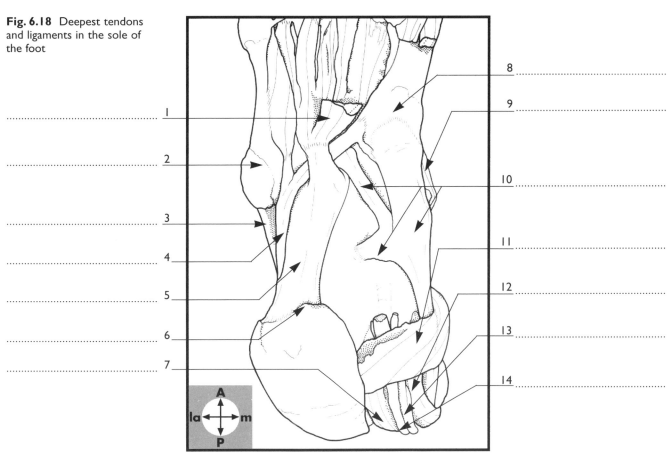

1 ....

2 ....

3 ....

4 ....

5 ....

6 ....

7 ....

8 ....

9 ....

10 ....

11 ....

12 ....

13 ....

14 ....

Fig. 6.19 Muscles and tendons in the anterior compartment of the leg and on dorsum of foot

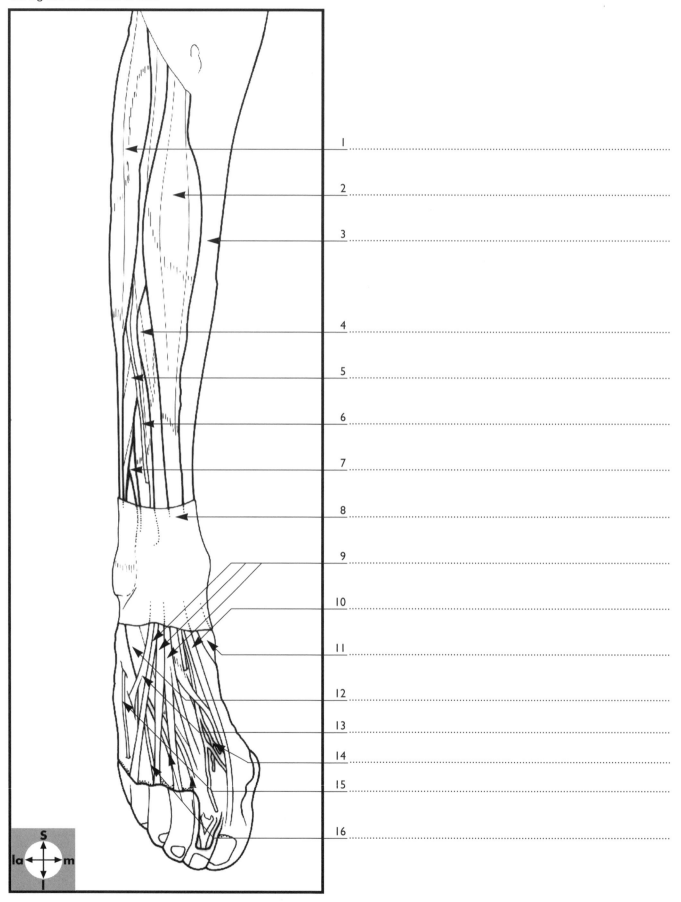

1 ....

2 ....

3 ....

4 ....

5 ....

6 ....

7 ....

8 ....

9 ....

10 ....

11 ....

12 ....

13 ....

14 ....

15 ....

16 ....

Fig. 6.20 Muscles, tendons and nerves in the anterior and lateral compartments of the leg

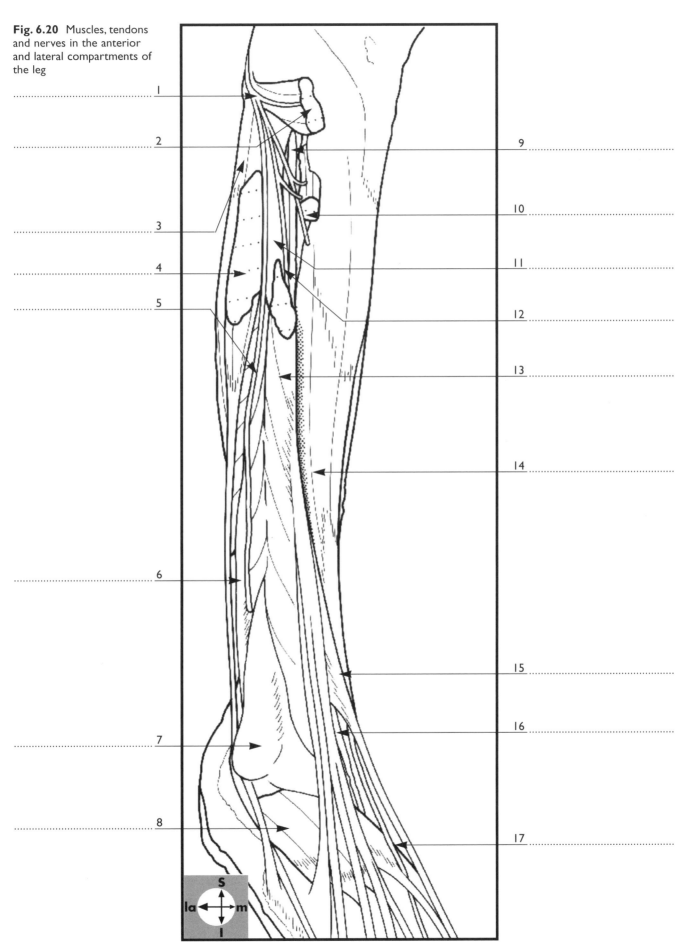

1

2

3

4

5

6

7

8

9

10

11

12

13

14

15

16

17

Fig. 6.21 Hip joint and related structures (anterior aspect)

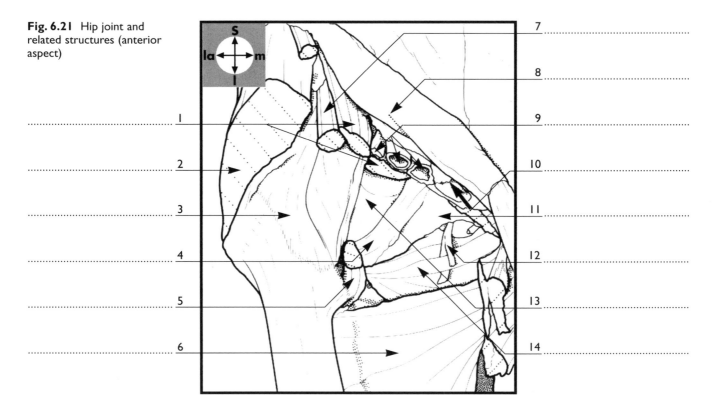

Fig. 6.22 Hip joint in coronal section showing internal structure and related structures

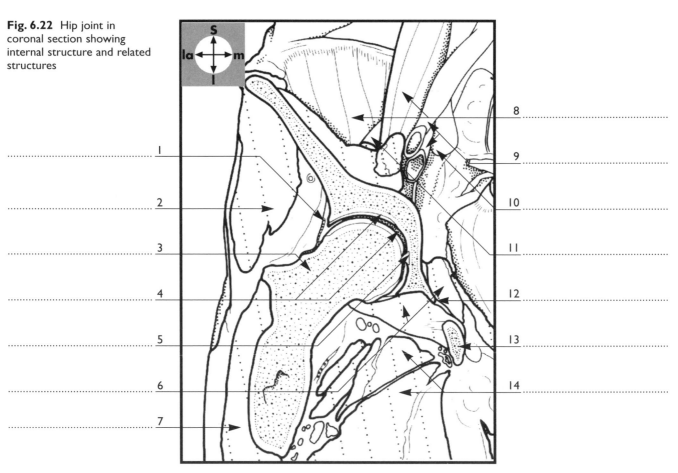

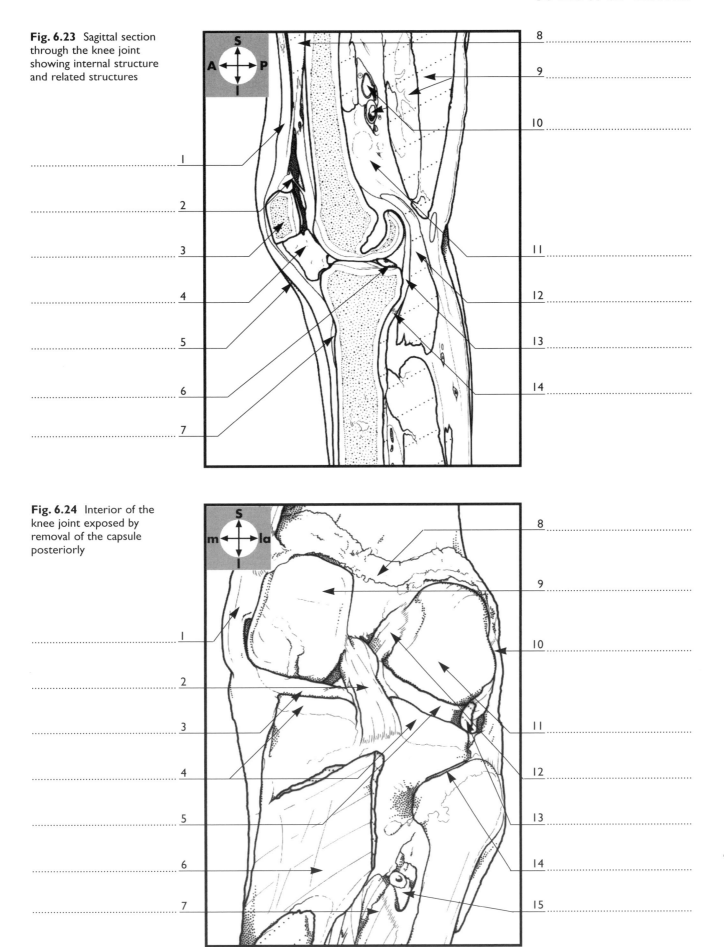

Fig. 6.23 Sagittal section through the knee joint showing internal structure and related structures

Fig. 6.24 Interior of the knee joint exposed by removal of the capsule posteriorly

Fig. 6.25 Ankle joint exposed to show associated ligaments
(lateral aspect)

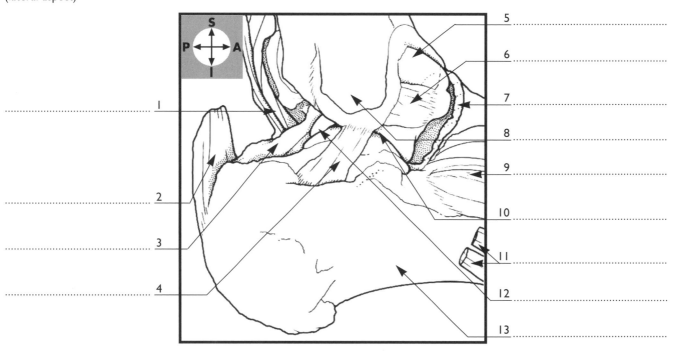

Fig. 6.26 Transverse section through the ankle (above joint)
showing related tendons, nerves and blood vessels

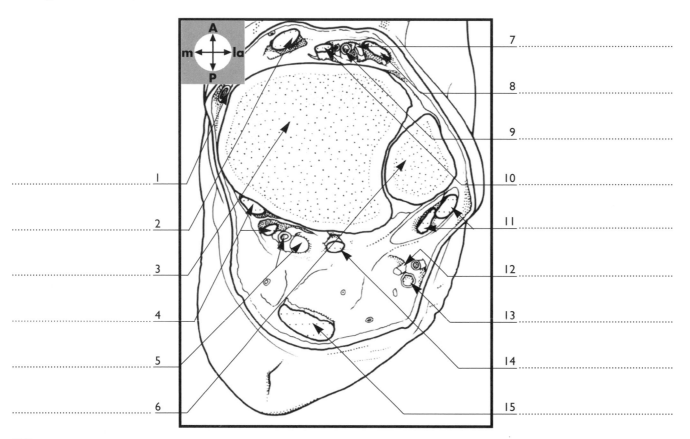

Fig. 6.27 Sagittal section through medial part of the foot
showing medial longitudinal arch and related structures

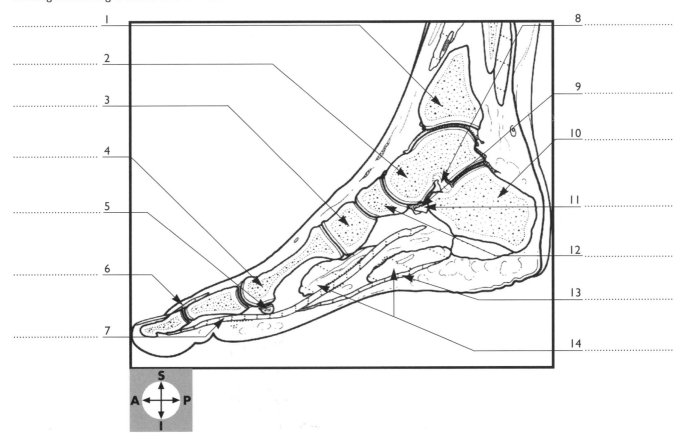

1

2

3

4

5

6

7

8

9

10

11

12

13

14

7. Head & Neck

Fig. 7.1 The main arteries of the head and neck

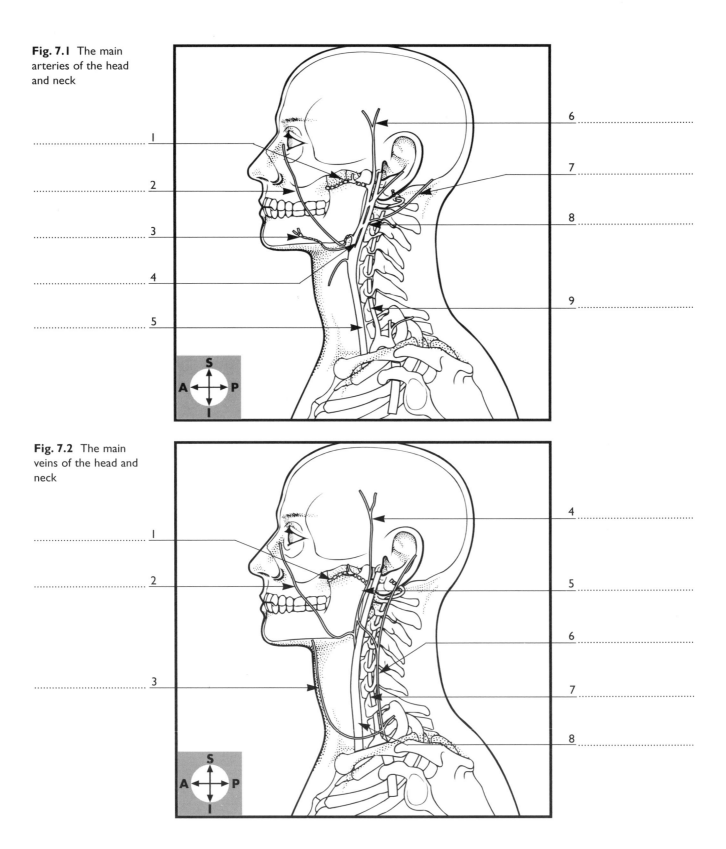

1
2
3
4
5

6
7
8
9

Fig. 7.2 The main veins of the head and neck

1
2

3

4

5

6

7

8

Fig. 7.3 Transverse section of the neck at the level of C4 showing the layers of cervical fascia

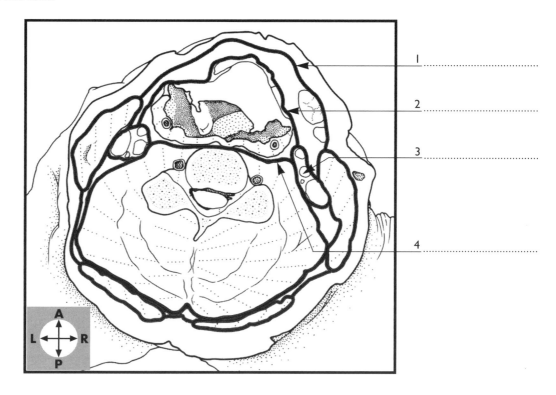

Fig. 7.4 The investing fascia and its enclosures

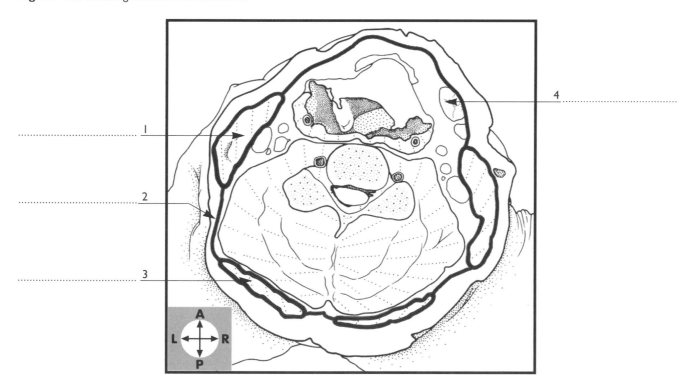

Fig. 7.5 The prevertebral fascia and its enclosures

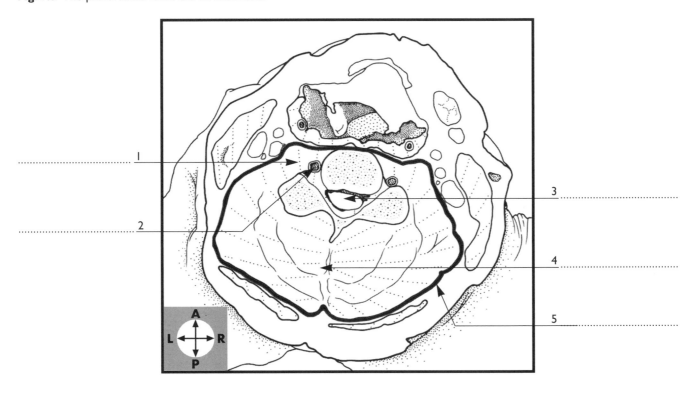

Fig. 7.6 The pretrachial fascia and carotid sheaths and their enclosures

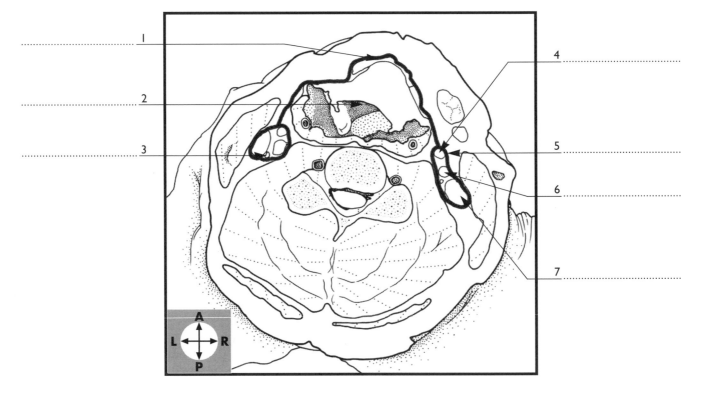

Fig. 7.7 Floor of the posterior triangle from which the prevertebral fascia has been removed

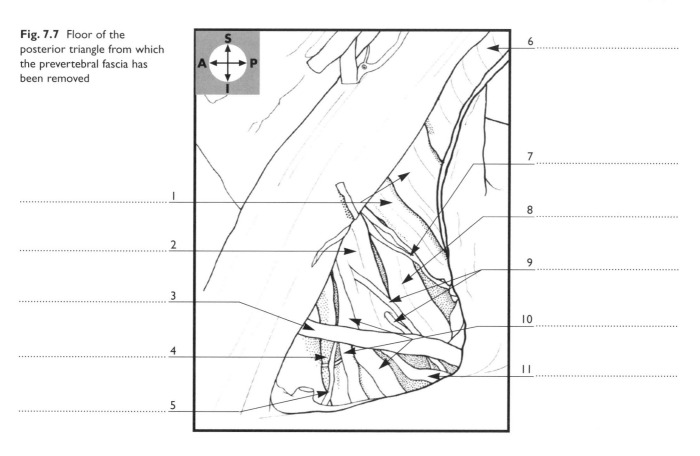

Fig. 7.8 Contents of the posterior triangle

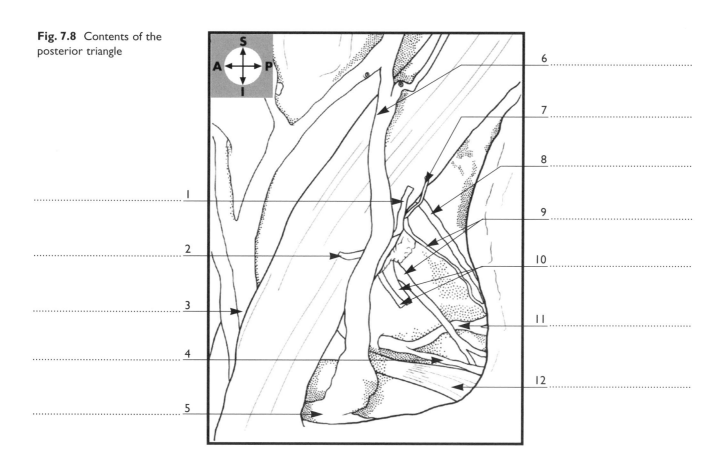

Fig. 7.9 The thyroid gland and its immediate blood supply revealed by removal of the pretracheal fascia

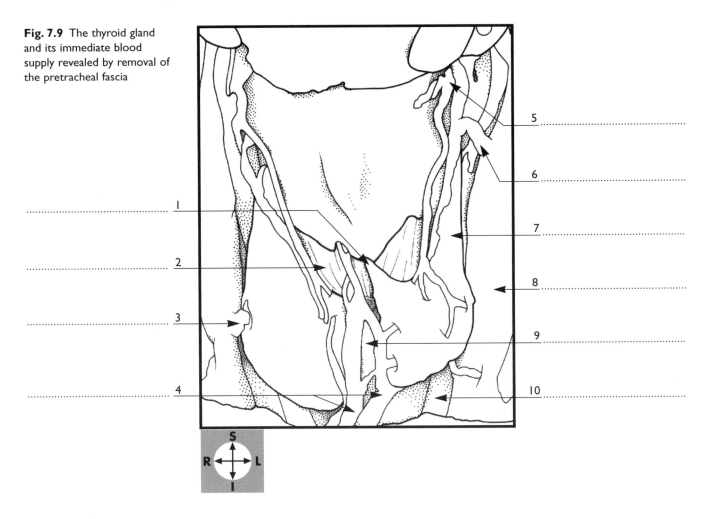

Fig. 7.10 The root of the neck

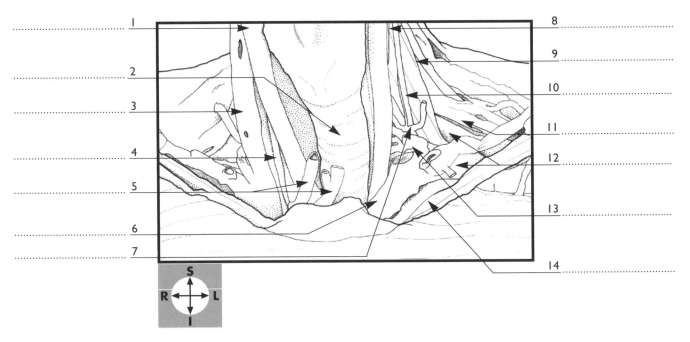

Fig. 7.11 Branches of the external carotid artery and the vagus, accessory and hypoglossal nerves

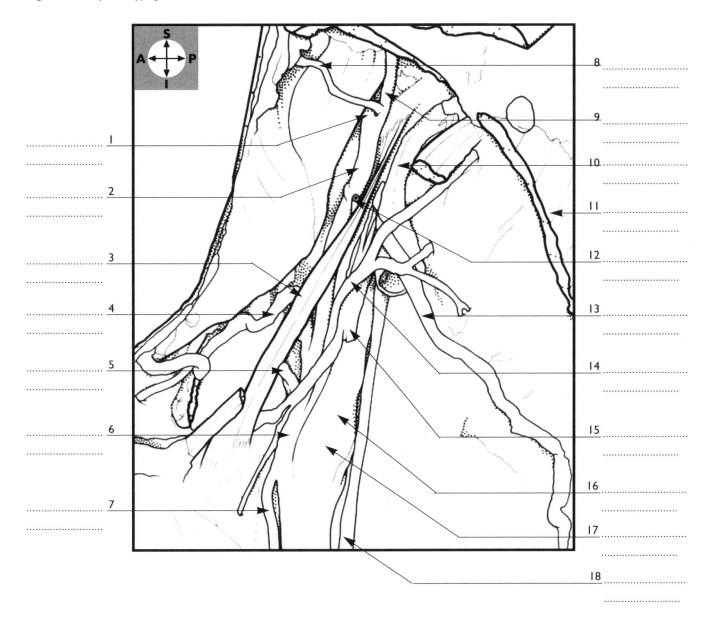

1 ....

2 ....

3 ....

4 ....

5 ....

6 ....

7 ....

8 ....

9 ....

10 ....

11 ....

12 ....

13 ....

14 ....

15 ....

16 ....

17 ....

18 ....

Fig. 7.12 The muscles of facial expression

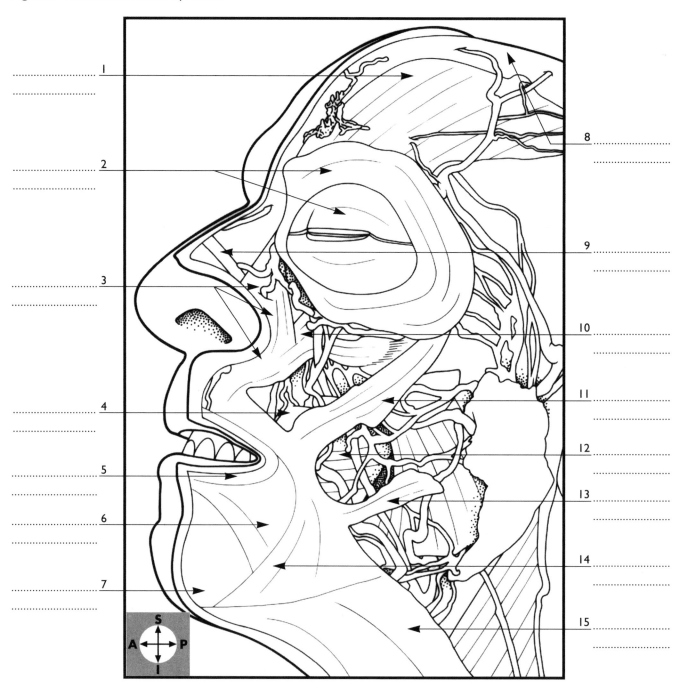

1 ....

2 ....

3 ....

4 ....

5 ....

6 ....

7 ....

8 ....

9 ....

10 ....

11 ....

12 ....

13 ....

14 ....

15 ....

Fig. 7.13 Temporalis

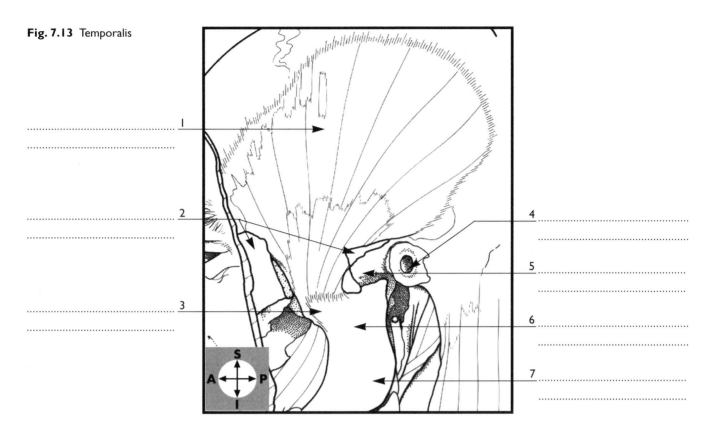

Fig. 7.14 Mandible

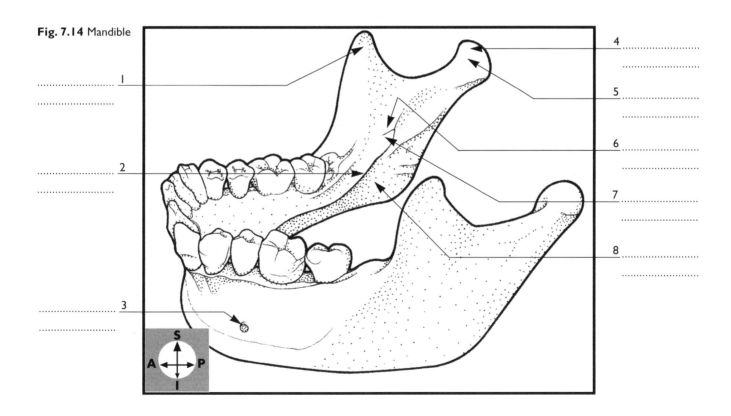

Fig. 7.15 Infratemporal fossa

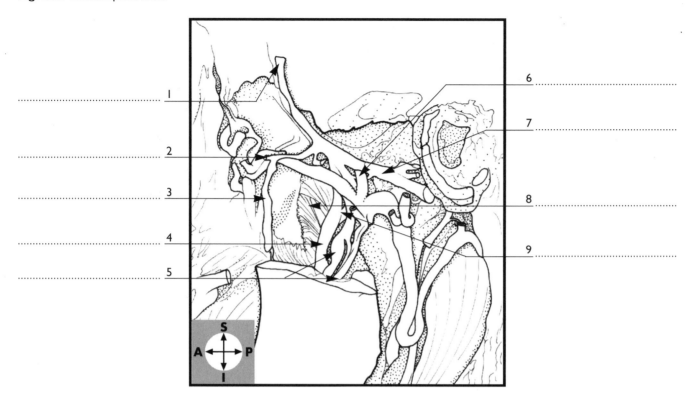

Fig. 7.16 Deeper structures in face seen after removal of part of the mandible

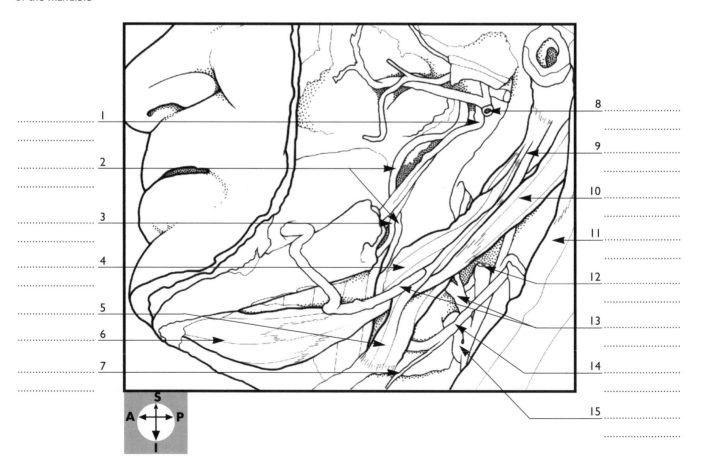

Fig. 7.17 Deep structures in the base of the tongue

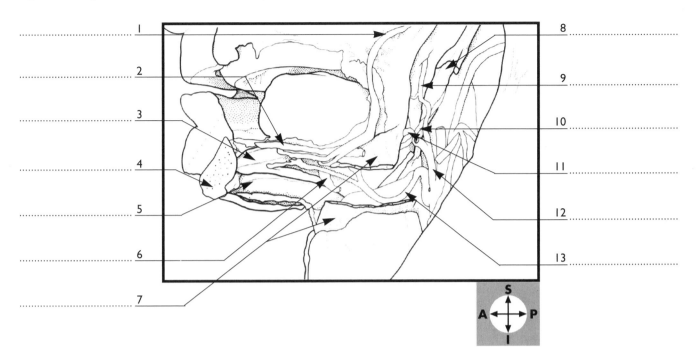

Fig. 7.18 Sagittal section through the tongue and surrounding structures

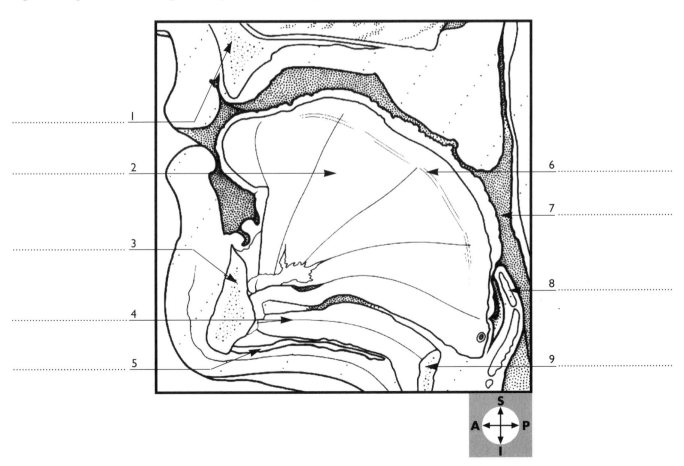

Fig. 7.19 Coronal section of the head

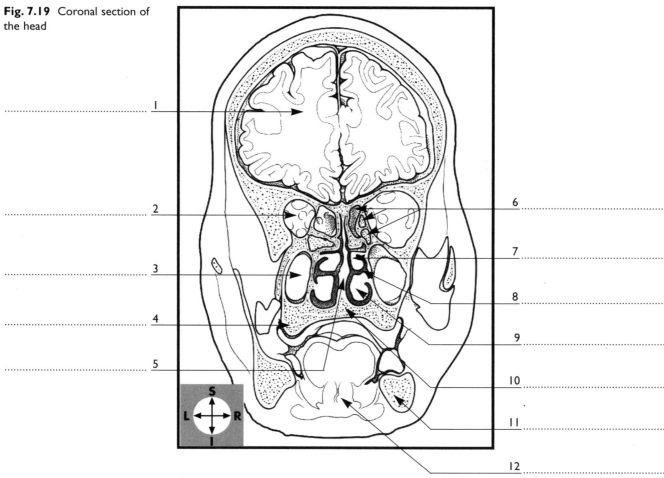

Fig. 7.20 Lateral wall of the nasal cavity

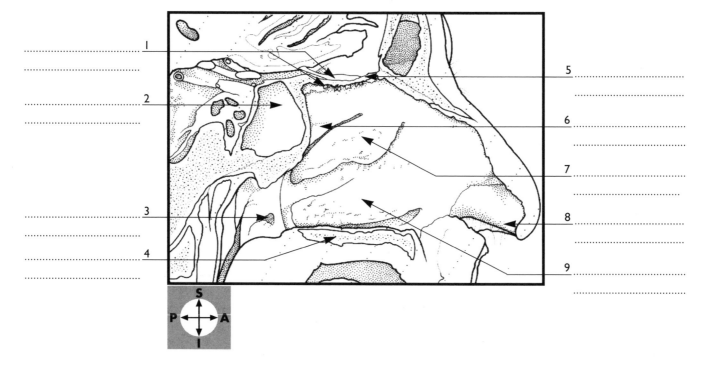

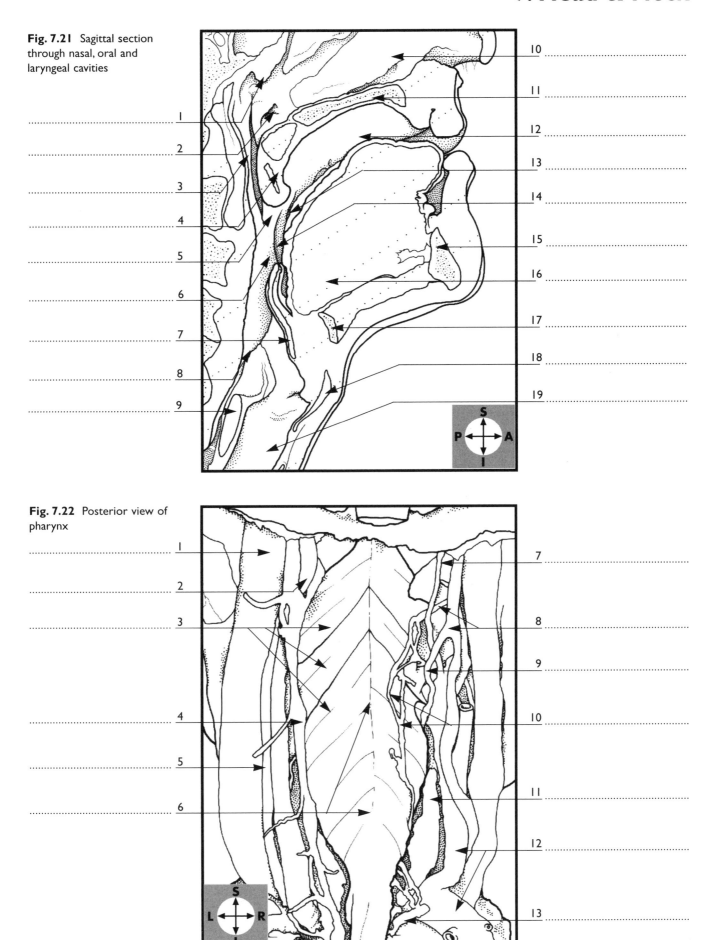

Fig. 7.21 Sagittal section through nasal, oral and laryngeal cavities

1
2
3
4
5
6
7
8
9

10
11
12
13
14
15
16
17
18
19

Fig. 7.22 Posterior view of pharynx

1
2
3
4
5
6

7
8
9
10
11
12
13

Fig. 7.23 The larynx

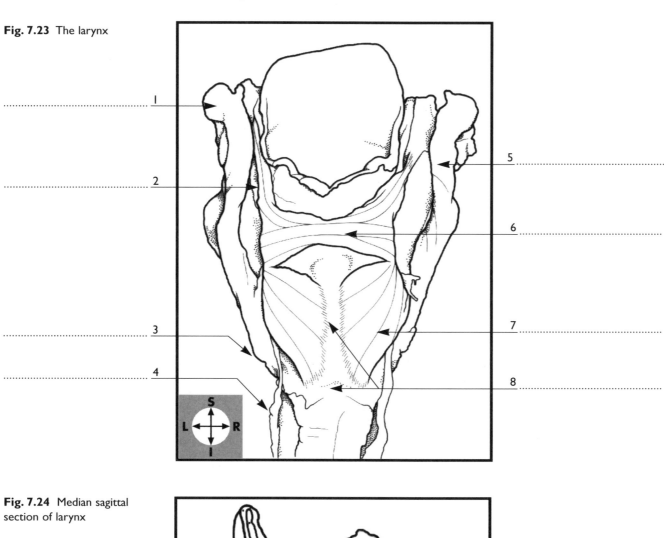

1
2
3
4
5
6
7
8

Fig. 7.24 Median sagittal
section of larynx

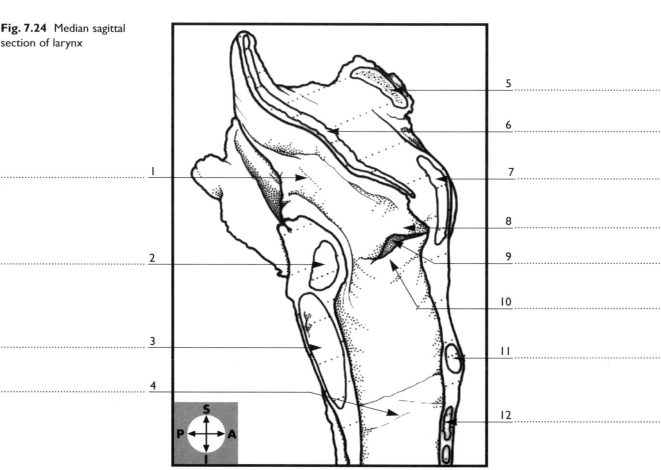

1
2
3
4
5
6
7
8
9
10
11
12

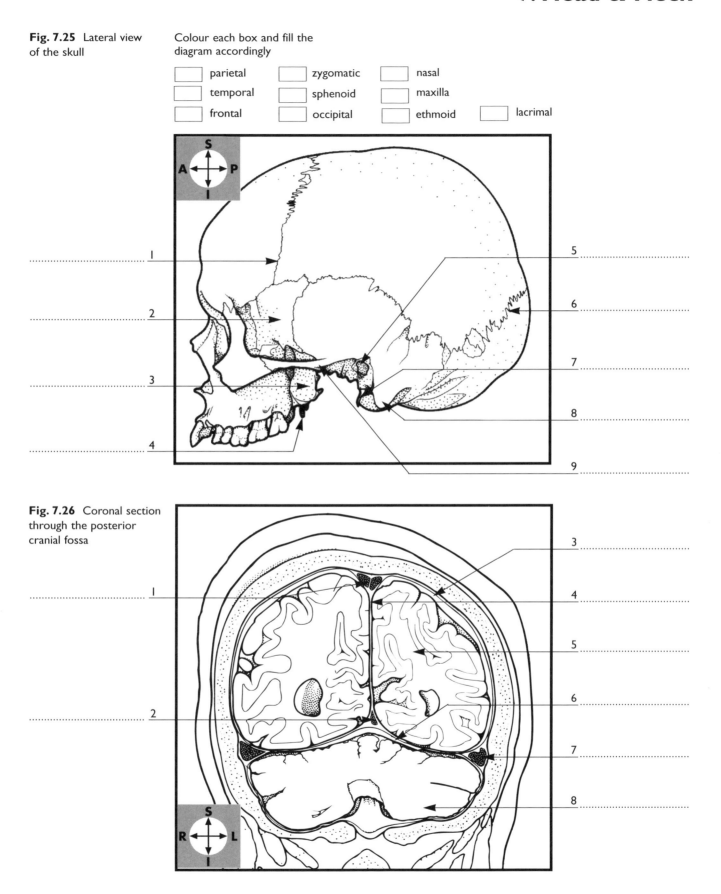

Fig. 7.25 Lateral view of the skull

Colour each box and fill the diagram accordingly

☐ parietal ☐ zygomatic ☐ nasal
☐ temporal ☐ sphenoid ☐ maxilla
☐ frontal ☐ occipital ☐ ethmoid ☐ lacrimal

Fig. 7.26 Coronal section through the posterior cranial fossa

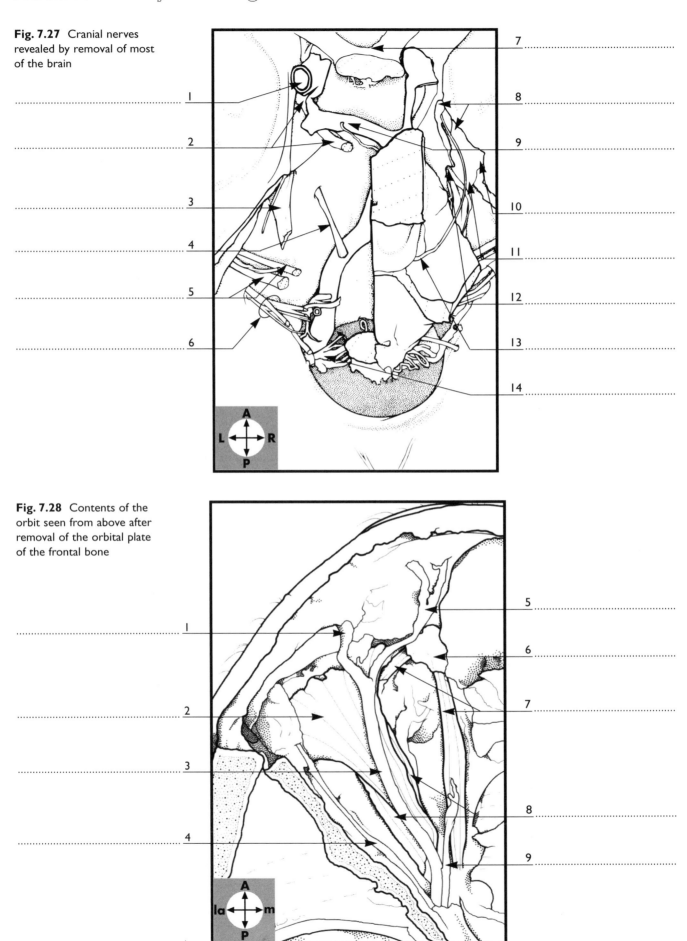

Fig. 7.27 Cranial nerves revealed by removal of most of the brain

Fig. 7.28 Contents of the orbit seen from above after removal of the orbital plate of the frontal bone

Fig. 7.29 Structures of the orbit seen following excision of superior rectus, levator palpebrae superioris and the superior division of the oculomotor nerve along with a quantity of orbital fat

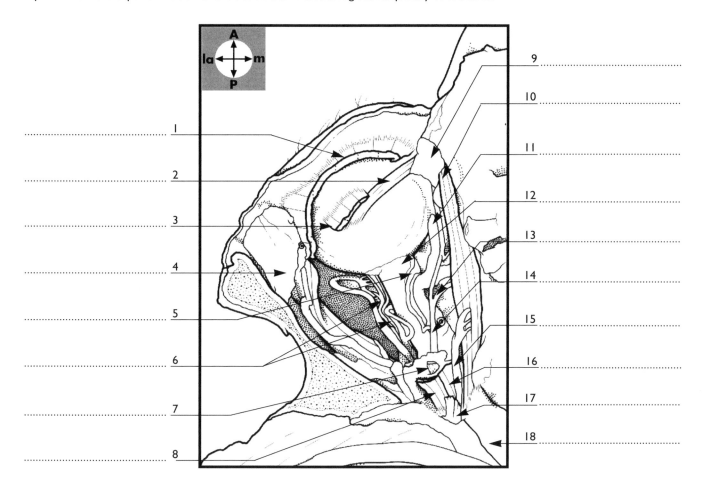

8. Back

Fig. 8.1 Superior view of a thoracic vertebra showing arrangement of the main groups of back muscles

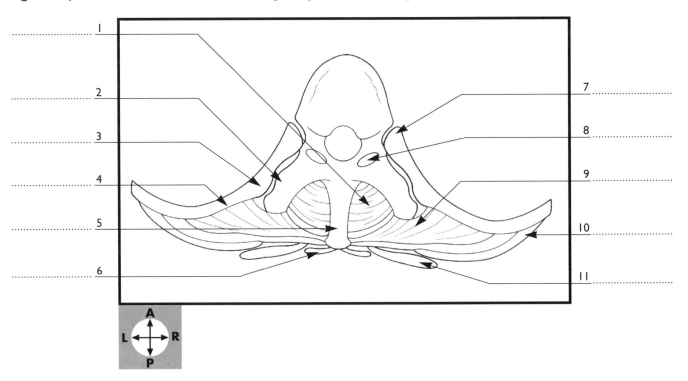

1 ....
2 ....
3 ....
4 ....
5 ....
6 ....

7 ....
8 ....
9 ....
10 ....
11 ....

Fig. 8.2 Superior view of a typical cervical vertebra showing spinal cord and a pair of spinal nerves

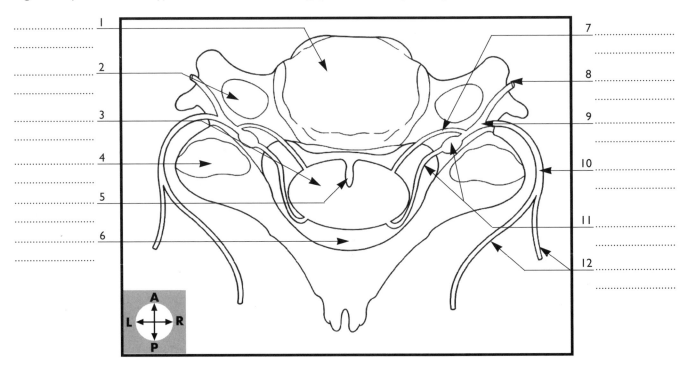

1 ....
2 ....
3 ....
4 ....
5 ....
6 ....

7 ....
8 ....
9 ....
10 ....
11 ....
12 ....

Fig. 8.3 Lateral view of a typical (fourth) cervical vertebra

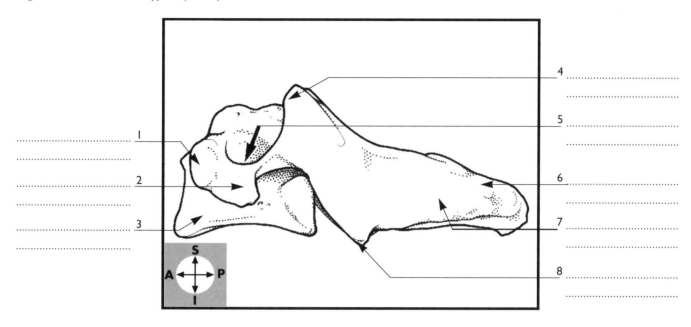

1 ....
2 ....
3 ....

4 ....
5 ....
6 ....
7 ....
8 ....

Fig. 8.4 Superior view of a typical (fourth) cervical vertebra

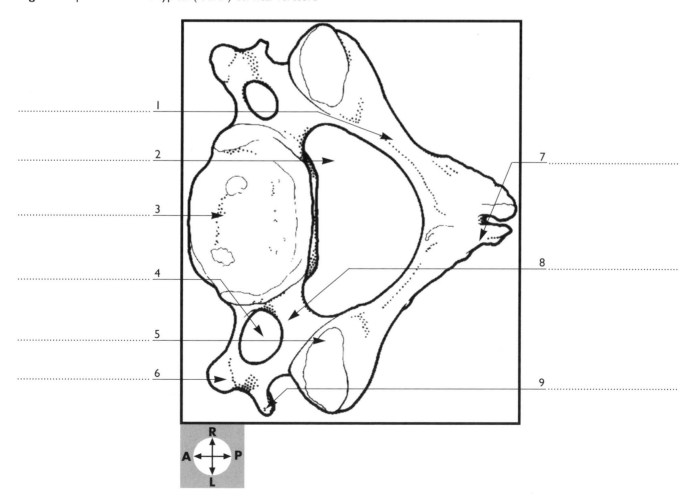

1 ....
2 ....
3 ....
4 ....
5 ....
6 ....

7 ....
8 ....
9 ....

Fig. 8.5 Base of the skull, atlas and axis in an expanded posterior view

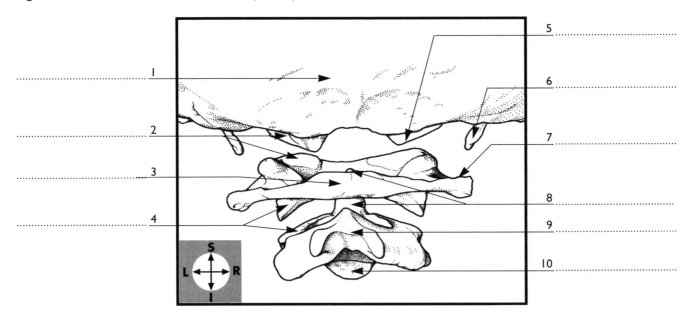

Fig. 8.6 Lateral views of the second and tenth thoracic vertebrae

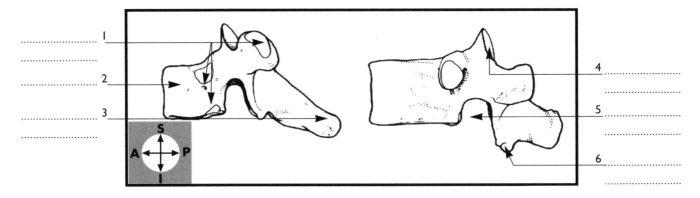

Fig. 8.7 Superior views of the second and tenth thoracic vertebrae

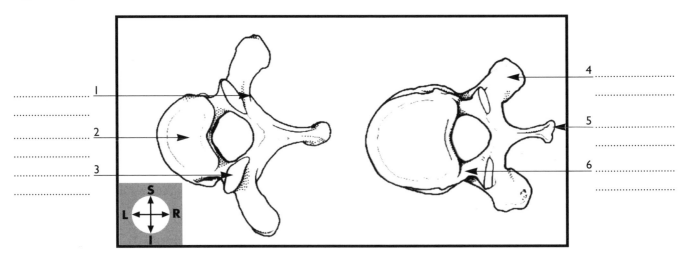

Fig. 8.8 Lateral view of a typical (third) lumbar vertebra

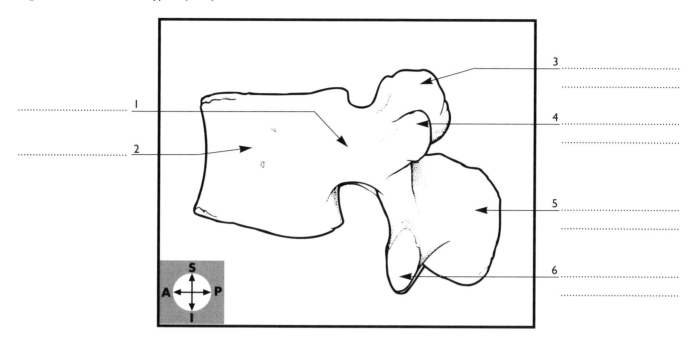

Fig. 8.9 Superior view of a typical (third) lumbar vertebra

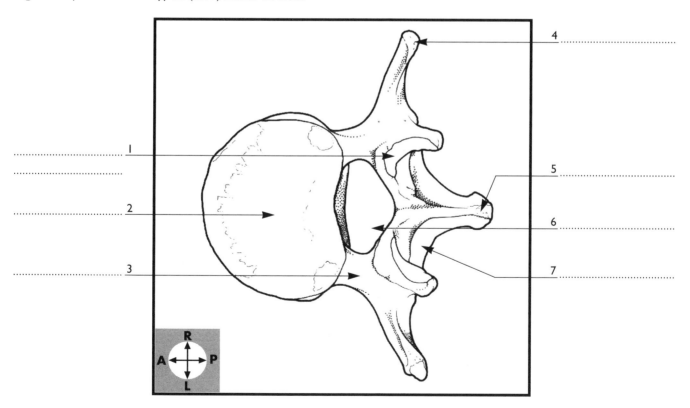

Fig. 8.10 Sagittal section of the lumbar vertebral column

Fig. 8.11 Back muscles exposed by removal of serratus posterior muscles, thoracolumbar fascia, and the upper limb girdle and its muscles

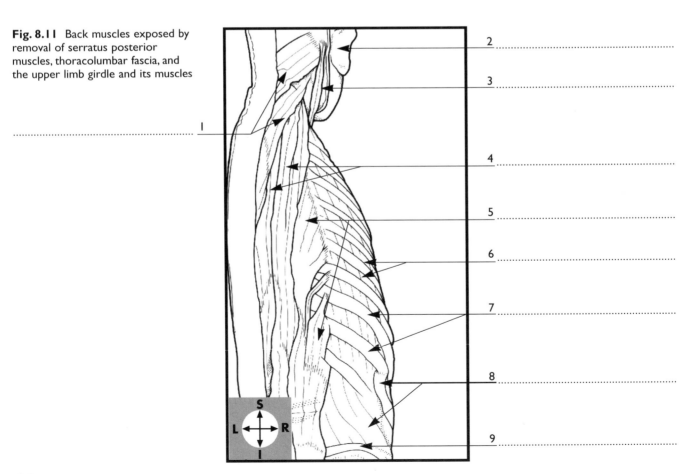

Fig. 8.12 Spinal meninges

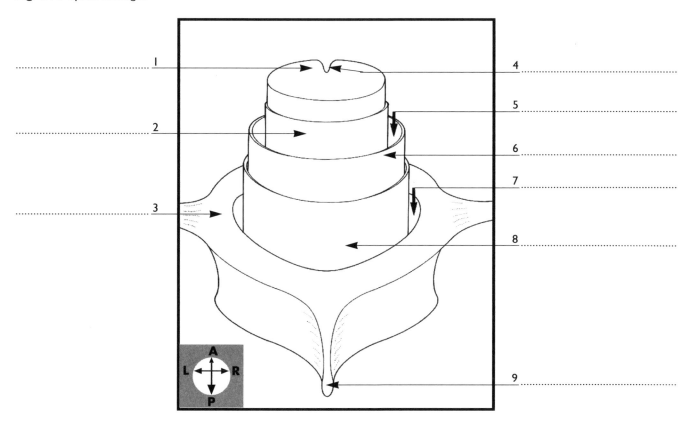

Fig. 8.13 Transverse section at the level of the second lumbar vertebra to show the back muscles and the contents of the vertebral foramen

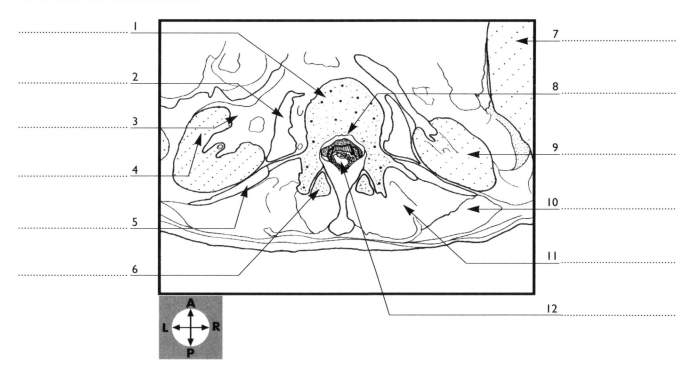

Answers

Chapter 1 Basic Anatomical Concepts

Fig. 1.1
1. frontal
2. temporal
3. zygomatic
4. mandible
5. first rib
6. manubrium
7. body of sternum
8. radius
9. ulna
10. hip bone
11. ilium
12. ischium
13. pubis
14. patella
15. tibia
16. fibula
17. maxilla
18. seventh cervical vertebra
19. first thoracic vertebra
20. lumbar vertebra
21. femur
22. tarsals
23. metatarsals
24. phalanges

Fig. 1.2
1. parietal
2. seventh cervical vertebra
3. first thoracic vertebra
4. pectoral girdle
5. clavicle
6. scapula
7. lumbar vertebra
8. phalanges
9. metacarpals
10. carpals
11. occipital
12. twelfth rib
13. sacrum
14. coccyx

Fig. 1.3
1. superficial temporal
2. maxillary
3. facial
4. lingual
5. superior thyroid
6. right common carotid
7. right vertebral
8. right subclavian
9. axillary
10. profunda brachii
11. brachial
12. radial
13. superficial palmar arch
14. interosseous
15. ulnar
16. femoral
17. popliteal
18. posterior tibial
19. anterior tibial
20. medial plantar
21. plantar arch

22. gonadal
23. abdominal aorta
24. posterior auricular
25. occipital
26. external carotid
27. internal carotid
28. left common carotid
29. left subclavian
30. brachiocephalic
31. right coronary
32. thoracic aorta
33. coeliac
34. renal
35. superior mesenteric
36. inferior mesenteric
37. common iliac
38. internal iliac
39. external iliac
40. profunda femoris
41. peroneal
42. lateral plantar
43. dorsalis pedis

Fig. 1.4
1. facial
2. right internal jugular
3. right vertebral
4. subclavian
5. right brachiocephalic
6. superior vena cava
7. hepatic
8. inferior vena cava
9. renal
10. gonadal
11. common iliac
12. external iliac
13. internal iliac
14. great saphenous
15. popliteal
16. short saphenous
17. dorsal arch
18. superficial temporal
19. left external jugular
20. left internal jugular
21. left brachiocephalic
22. axillary
23. cephalic
24. basilic
25. venae comitantes
26. dorsal arch
27. femoral
28. venae comitantes

Fig. 1.5
1. median
2. ulnar
3. radial
4. musculocutaneous
5. first lumbar
6. femoral
7. obturator
8. sciatic
9. common peroneal
10. tibial
11. saphenous
12. deep peroneal
13. medial plantar

14. first cervical
15. cervical plexus (C2–C4)
16. brachial plexus (C5–T1)
17. T2–T12
18. lumbar plexus (L1–L4)
19. sacral plexus (L4–S4)
20. fifth sacral & first coccygeal
21. superficial peroneal
22. lateral plantar

Chapter 2 Thorax

Fig. 2.1
1. first rib
2. manubrium
3. body of sternum
4. costal margin
5. intervertebral disc
6. first thoracic vertebra
7. second rib
8. costal cartilage
9. xiphoid process
10. twelfth rib

Fig. 2.2
1. external intercostal muscle
2. internal intercostal muscle
3. parietal pleura
4. internal intercostal muscles (cut)
5. innermost intercostal muscles
6. intercostal artery
7. internal intercostal muscle (cut)
8. external intercostal muscle (cut)
9. intercostal nerve

Fig. 2.3
1. right & left brachiocephalic veins
2. internal thoracic vessels
3. mediastinum
4. musculophrenic vessels
5. left subclavian artery vessels
6. second rib
7. third intercostal nerve
8. parietal pleura
9. inferior border of left lung
10. costodiaphragmatic recess
11. costal margin

Fig. 2.4
1. brachiocephalic trunk
2. right brachiocephalic vein
3. horizontal fissure
4. diaphragm
5. left common carotid artery
6. left brachiocephalic vein
7. fibrous pericardium
8. lingula

Fig. 2.5
1. right & left phrenic nerves
2. right atrial appendage
3. ascending aorta
4. pulmonary trunk
5. pericardial cavity
6. fibrous pericardium (cut)
7. visceral serous pericardium

Fig. 2.6
1. right pulmonary artery
2. pulmonary veins
3. right atrial appendage
4. fossa ovalis
5. valve & inferior vena cava
6. superior vena cava
7. aortic sinuses
8. crista terminalis (cut)
9. musculi pectinati
10. orifice of coronary sinus

Fig. 2.7
1. anterior interventricular artery
2. pulmonary sinus & valve
3. left coronary artery
4. pulmonary vein
5. right ventricle
6. right coronary artery
7. aortic valve
8. position of transverse pericardial sinus
9. superior vena cava
10. left atrium

Fig. 2.8
1. pulmonary trunk
2. anterior interventricular artery
3. mitral valve & chordae tendineae
4. papillary muscle
5. trabeculae carneae
6. ascending aorta
7. circumflex artery
8. coronary sinus (cut)

Fig. 2.9
1. anterior interventricular artery
2. right ventricular wall
3. papillary muscle
4. left ventricular wall
5. marginal artery
6. trabeculae carneae
7. interventricular septum

Fig. 2.10
1. arch of aorta
2. left pulmonary artery
3. pulmonary trunk
4. infundibulum of right ventricle
5. mitral valve

6. muscular & membranous parts of interventricular septum (cut)
7. tricuspid valve
8. left vagus nerve
9. left recurrent laryngeal nerve
10. ligamentum arteriosum
11. anterior interventricular artery (cut)
12. papillary muscles
13. left ventricular wall
14. right ventricular wall

Fig. 2.11
1. ascending aorta
2. pulmonary trunk
3. anterior cardiac veins
4. right coronary artery
5. anterior atrioventricular groove
6. marginal artery
7. left phrenic nerve
8. great cardiac vein
9. fibrous pericardium
10. ventricular branch of left coronary artery
11. anterior interventricular artery

Fig. 2.12
1. ascending aorta
2. pulmonary trunk
3. anterior interventricular artery
4. ventricular branches of left coronary artery
5. superior vena cava
6. left coronary artery
7. left atrial appendage (displaced)
8. circumflex artery
9. coronary sinus (cut)

Fig. 2.13
1. left atrial appendage
2. great cardiac vein
3. ventricular branch of left coronary artery
4. posterior vein of left ventricle
5. left pulmonary veins
6. oblique vein of left atrium
7. atrioventricular groove
8. coronary sinus

Fig. 2.14
1. left & right brachioc- ephalic veins
2. vagal & sympathetic cardiac nerves
3. ligamentum arteriosum
4. left phrenic nerve
5. fibrous pericardium
6. inferior thyroid vein
7. left superior intercostal vein
8. aortic arch
9. left vagus nerve
10. left pulmonary artery (cut)
11. left bronchus (cut)
12. pulmonary veins (cut)

Fig. 2.15
1. left common carotid artery
2. left atrial appendage
3. pulmonary trunk
4. fibrous pericardium (cut)
5. left subclavian artery
6. left vagus nerve
7. left phrenic nerve
8. left lung root
9. diaphragm

Fig. 2.16
1. right vagus nerve
2. azygos vein (cut)
3. parietal pleura (cut)
4. azygos vein (cut)
5. inferior vena cava (cut)
6. trachea (cut)
7. left recurrent laryngeal nerve
8. left vagus nerve
9. descending aorta
10. thoracic duct
11. oesophagus & plexus

Fig. 2.17
1. right superior intercostal vein
2. right sympathetic trunk
3. innermost intercostal muscles
4. posterior intercostal vein & artery
5. intercostal nerve
6. thoracic duct
7. azygos vein
8. descending aorta

Fig. 2.18
1. thoracic duct
2. azygos vein
3. accessory hemiazygos vein
4. ramus communicans
5. posterior intercostal arteries (cut)
6. descending aorta (cut)
7. left sympathetic trunk
8. posterior intercostal vein & artery
9. intercostal nerve
10. greater splanchnic nerve
11. hemiazygos vein

Chapter 3   Upper Limb

Fig. 3.1
1. supraclavicular nerves
cutaneous nerves of arm:
2. upper lateral
3. lower lateral
4. posterior
5. medial
cutaneous nerves of forearm:
6. lateral
7. posterior
8. medial

Fig. 3.2
1. subclavian
2. thoracoacromial
3. axillary
4. subscapular
5. profunda brachii

6. collateral
7. brachial
8. ulnar
9. radial
10. interosseous
11. deep palmar arch
12. superficial palmar arch

Fig. 3.3
1. subclavian
2. cephalic
3. axillary
4. venae comitantes of brachial artery
5. venae comitantes
6. basilic
7. dorsal venous arch

Fig. 3.4
1. lateral cord
2. medial cord
3. median nerve
4. anterior interosseous nerve

Fig. 3.5
1. lateral cord of brachial plexus
2. medial cord of brachial plexus
3. musculocutaneous nerve
4. ulnar nerve
5. lateral cutaneous nerve of forearm
6. dorsal branch of ulnar nerve
7. palmar branch of ulnar nerve

Fig. 3.6
1. posterior cord of brachial plexus
2. axillary nerve
3. radial nerve
4. posterior interosseous nerve
5. superficial branch of radial nerve
6. digital branches of radial nerve

Fig. 3.7
1. scapula
2. teres minor
3. deltoid
4. tendon of triceps long head
5. axillary vein & artery
6. shaft of humerus
7. tendon of biceps long head
8. cephalic vein
9. infraspinatus
10. subscapularis
11. thoracic cavity
12. intercostal muscle
13. rib
14. serratus anterior
15. coracobrachialis & biceps short head
16. pectoralis minor
17. pectoralis major

Fig. 3.8
1. coracoid process
2. coracobrachialis

3. lower trunk (cut)
4. biceps long head
5. circumflex humeral arteries
6. subscapular artery
7. latissimus dorsi overlying teres major
8. profunda brachii artery
9. brachial artery
10. upper trunk (cut)
11. subclavian artery
12. middle trunk (cut)
13. scalenus anterior
14. posterior cord
15. subscapularis
16. axillary nerve
17. radial nerve
18. thoracodorsal nerve
19. long thoracic nerve
20. serratus anterior
21. circumflex scapular artery

Fig. 3.9
1. lateral pectoral
2. lateral head of median
3. radial
4. axillary
5. musculocutaneous
6. suprascapular
7. dorsal scapular
8. subclavian
9. medial head of median
10. long thoracic
11. medial pectoral
12. medial cutaneous of arm (brachial)
13. medial cutaneous of forearm (antebrachial)
14. ulnar
15. median
a) upper subscapulor
b) thoracoclorsal
c) lower subscapular

Fig. 3.10
1. deltoid (cut)
2. tendons of short & long heads
3. biceps brachii
4. brachioradialis
5. lateral cutaneous nerve of forearm
6. coracoid process
7. clavicle
8. axillary vein
9. coracobrachialis
10. pectoralis minor (cut)
11. median nerve
12. latissimus dorsi
13. medial cutaneous nerve of forearm
14. aponeurosis of biceps

Fig. 3.11
1. basilic vein
2. medial head of triceps
3. biceps brachii
4. brachial artery & venae comitantes
5. aponeurosis of biceps
6. lateral cutaneous nerve of forearm
7. tendon of biceps
8. median nerve
9. brachioradialis

10. pronator teres
11. radial artery & vena comitans

Fig. 3.12
1. brachioradialis (cut)
2. fused tendons of superficial flexors (cut)
3. tendon of biceps (cut)
4. supinator
5. flexor pollicis longus
6. flexor digitorum profundus
7. tendon of brachioradialis
8. tendon of flexor carpi ulnaris (cut)
9. tendon of flexor carpi radialis (cut)
10. lumbricals
11. tendons of flexor digitorum superficialis

Fig. 3.13
1. medial supracondylar ridge
2. common flexor origin
3. coronoid process of ulna
4. head
5. neck
6. brachialis
7. tuberosity of radius (biceps)
8. supinator
9. pronator teres
10. flexor digitorum profundus
11. flexor pollicis longus
12. pronator quadratus
13. head of ulna
14. brachioradialis
15 styloid processes

Fig. 3.14
1. vena comitans & brachial artery
2. radial nerve
3. median nerve
4. extensor carpi radialis longus
5. deep head of pronator teres
6. flexor carpi ulnaris (cut)
7. common interosseous artery
8. posterior interosseous artery
9. anterior interosseous nerve
10. anterior interosseous artery
11. ulnar nerve
12. ulnar artery
13. flexor digitorum profundus
14. radial artery
15. flexor pollicis longus
16. median nerve
17. superficial radial nerve
18. flexor digitorum superficialis tendons (cut)
19. flexor carpi radialis tendon (cut)
20. flexor retinaculum

Fig. 3.15
1. digital nerves
2. fibrous flexor sheaths
3. abductor digiti minimi
4. palmaris brevis
5. flexor retinaculum
6. ulnar nerve & artery
7. first dorsal interosseous
8. palmar aponeurosis
9. adductor pollicis
10. abductor pollicis brevis
11. abductor pollicis longus
12. median nerve
13. tendon of palmaris longus

Fig. 3.16
1. tendon of flexor digitorum superficialis
2. digital artery
3. tendon of flexor digitorum profundus
4. digital vein
5. skin crease
6. digital nerve
7. fibrous flexor sheath
8. proximal phalanx
9. extensor expansion

Fig. 3.17
1. tendons of flexor digitorum profundus
2. tendons of flexor digitorum superficialis (cut)
3. lumbrical muscles
4. tendon of flexor digitorum superficialis
5. fibrous flexor sheath (cut)
6. adductor pollicis
7. flexor pollicis longus

Fig. 3.18
1. digital arteries
2. digital branches of ulnar nerve
3. superficial palmar arch
4. opponens digiti minimi
5. ulnar nerve & artery
6. median nerve
7. flexor carpi ulnaris tendon
8. digital branches of median nerve
9. recurrent branch of median nerve
10. flexor pollicis brevis
11. abductor pollicis brevis
12. flexor retinaculum
13. vena comitans & radial artery
14. tendon of flexor carpi radialis
15. flexor digitorum superficialis

Fig. 3.19
1. metacarpal arteries
2. flexor digiti minimi brevis
3. deep branch of ulnar nerve
4. flexor retinaculum (cut)
5. ulnar nerve
6. first dorsal interosseous muscle
7. interossei
8. adductor pollicis (cut)

9. deep palmar arch
10. radial artery

Fig. 3.20
1. splenius capitis
2. left trapezius
3. right trapezius
4. rhomboid major
5 deltoid
6. fascia overlying infraspinatus
7. teres major
8. latissimus dorsi
9. spinous processes

Fig. 3.21
1. supraspinatus
2. coracoid process
3. tendon of biceps brachii
4. lesser tubercle of humerus
5 tendon of long head of biceps
6. tendon of teres major
7. brachialis
8. superior angle of scapula
9. suprascapular ligament
10. medial border of scapula
11. subscapularis
12. tendon of latissimus dorsi
13. inferior angle of scapula

Fig. 3.22
1. quadrilateral space
2. infraspinatus
3. long head of triceps
4. teres minor
5. axillary nerve
6. teres major
7. triangular intermuscular space
8. radial nerve
9. lateral head of triceps

Fig. 3.23
1. common extensor origin
2. medial epicondyle
3. anconeus
4. extensor digitorum
5. flexor carpi ulnaris
6. extensor carpi radialis longus
7. extensor carpi ulnaris
8. abductor pollicis longus
9. radius
10. ulna
11. extensor carpi radialis brevis & longus
12. extensor pollicis longus
13. extensor digiti minimi
14. first dorsal interosseous
15. extensor digitorum
16. extensor indicis

Fig. 3.24
1. brachialis
2. radial nerve
3. biceps tendon (cut)
4. brachioradialis
5. flexor carpi radialis
6. extensor carpi radialis longus tendon
7. radial artery
8. abductor pollicis longus tendon (cut)
9. thenar muscles
10. hypothenar muscles

Fig. 3.25
1. supinator
2. brachioradialis
3. extensor carpi radialis brevis
4. subcutaneous border of ulna
5. abductor pollicis longus & tendon
6. extensor pollicis brevis & tendon
7. dorsal tubercle of radius
8. extensor indicis
9. extensor carpi radialis brevis
10. extensor carpi radialis longus
11. radial artery
12. extensor pollicis longus

Fig. 3.26
1. first dorsal interosseous muscle
2. extensor indicis
3 extensor digitorum
4. extensor pollicis longus
5. extensor pollicis brevis
6 extensor hoods
7. intertendinous connection
8. abductor digiti minimi
9. extensor digiti minimi
10. extensor retinaculum
11. extensor carpi ulnaris

Fig. 3.27
1. pectoralis major
2. clavicle
3. subclavius
4. axillary artery
5. axillary fat
6. thoracic cavity
7. blade of scapula
8. serratus anterior
9. subscapularis
10. head of humerus
11. glenoid surface
12. glenoid labrum
13. deltoid
14. infraspinatus

Fig. 3.28
1. supraspinatus (cut)
2. scapular spine (cut)
3. vertebral border of scapula
4. infraspinatus (cut)
5. long head of triceps (cut)
6. teres minor (cut)
7. coracoid process
8. joint capsule
9. rotator cuff
10. surgical neck of humerus
11. shaft of humerus

Fig. 3.29
1. fat pad in olecranon fossa
2. subcutaneous fat
3. triceps brachii
4. humerus
5. olecranon & bursa
6. articular cartilage
7. head of radius
8. biceps brachii
9. brachialis

Answers

10. capsule of elbow joint
11. brachioradialis
12. annular ligament
13. radial nerve
14. supinator

Fig. 3.30
1. ulnar artery & nerve
2. hypothenar muscles
3. flexor retinaculum
4. pisiform
5. digital flexor tendons
6. articular cartilage
7. digital extensor tendons
8. median nerve
9. thenar muscles
10. flexor carpi radialis
11. trapezium
12. flexor pollicis longus
13. radial artery

Fig. 3.31
1. ulnar nerve
2. ulnar artery
3. flexor carpi ulnaris (cut)
4. flexor digitorum superficialis
5. ulnar nerve
6. flexor digitorum profundus
7. superficial palmar arch
8. thenar muscles
9. flexor retinaculum
10. flexor carpi radialis (cut)
11. median nerve
12. flexor pollicis longus
13. radial artery & nerve

Chapter 4   Abdomen

Fig. 4.1
1. liver
2. gall bladder
3. ascending colon
4. caecum & appendix
5. ileum (cut)
6. stomach
7. pancreas
8. transverse colon (cut)
9. jejunum (cut)
10. duodenum
11. sigmoid colon

Fig. 4.2
1. suprarenal gland
2. spleen
3. kidney
4. ureter
5. bladder

Fig. 4.3
1. coeliac
2. superior mesenteric
3. abdominal aorta
4. common iliac
5. femoral
6. diaphragm
7. renal
8. gonadal arteries
9. inferior mesenteric
10. external iliac
11. internal iliac

Fig. 4.4
1. hepatic

2. gonadal
3. inferior vena cava
4. external iliac
5. renal
6. common iliac
7. internal iliac
8. femoral

Fig. 4.5
1. liver
2. portal
3. superior mesenteric
4. spleen
5. splenic
6. inferior mesenteric

Fig. 4.6
1. external oblique (cut)
2. rectus abdominis & tendinous intersection
3. pyramidalis
4. intercostal nerves
5. transversus abdominis & aponeurosis
6. inferior epigastric vessels
7. ilioinguinal nerve (cut)

Fig. 4.7
1. deep inguinal ring
2. pubic symphysis & crest
3. root of penis
4. inguinal ligament & anterior superior iliac spine
5. superficial inguinal ring
6. pubic tubercle
7. spermatic cord

Fig. 4.8
1. external oblique aponeurosis (cut)
2. internal oblique (cut)
3. conjoint tendon
4. vas deferens
5. lacunar ligament
6. pubic tubercle
7. transversus abdominis
8. transversalis fascia
9. internal spermatic fascia
10. testicular veins & artery
11. pampiniform plexus
12. testicular artery

Fig. 4.9
1. testis & tunica albuginea
2. parietal layer of tunica vaginalis
3. vas deferens
4. epididymis
5. visceral layer of tunica vaginalis
6. external spermatic fascia

Fig 4.10
1. parietal peritoneum
2. aorta
3. fourth part of duodenum
4. splenic flexure of colon
5. peritoneum covering retroperitoneal structures
6. inferior vena cava & right renal vein
7. superior mesenteric vessels
8. head of pancreas

9. second part of duodenum
10. liver
11. right kidney

Fig. 4.11
1. superior pole of right kidney
2. right suprarenal gland
3. liver
4. inferior vena cava
5. opening into lesser sac
6. portal vein
7. spleen
8. left suprarenal gland
9. splenorenal ligament
10. aorta & coeliac trunk
11. gastrosplenic ligament
12. greater curve of stomach
13. lesser omentum & lesser curve of stomach

Fig. 4.12
1. inferior vena cava (cut)
2. oesophagus
3. liver (cut)
4. lesser omentum
5. anterior surface of stomach
6. aorta
7. left dome of diaphragm (cut)
8. gastrosplenic ligament
9. spleen
10. right gastroepiploic artery
11. transverse mesocolon

Fig. 4.13
1. spleen
2. oesophagus (cut)
3. splenic artery & vein
4. left renal vein
5. fourth part of duodenum (cut)
6. tail of pancreas
7. left kidney
8. inferior mesenteric vein
9. colon (cut)

Fig. 4.14
1. neck of pancreas
2. hepatic artery
3. gastroduodenal artery
4. second part of duodenum
5. superior mesenteric artery & vein
6. head of pancreas
7. body of pancreas
8. spleen
9. tail of pancreas
10. left kidney
11. splenic vein
12. uncinate process
13. third part of duodenum

Fig. 4.15
1. caudate lobe
2. portal vein
3. hepatic artery
4. quadrate lobe
5. fissure & round ligament
6. bare area
7. hepatic ducts
8. indentation for right kidney
9. gall bladder

Fig. 4.16
1. posterior surface of stomach
2. coeliac trunk (cut)
3. splenic artery (cut)
4. body of pancreas (cut)
5. splenic vein (cut)
6. inferior mesenteric vein
7. superior mesenteric artery (cut) & vein
8. aorta (cut)
9. lesser omentum
10. caudate lobe
11. inferior vena cava (cut)
12. bare area of liver
13. portal vein
14. right kidney
15. bile duct
16. duodenum

Fig. 4.17
1. caudate lobe of liver
2. portal vein
3. left & right branches of hepatic artery
4. bile duct
5. cystic duct
6. round ligament (cut)
7. first part of duodenum
8. left gastric artery & vein
9. pancreas
10. stomach
11. gastroduodenal artery
12. right gastric artery

Fig. 4.18
1. greater omentum (reflected)
2. transverse colon
3. mesentery of small intestine
4. ileum
5. caecum
6. jejunum
7. sigmoid colon
8. bladder

Fig. 4.19
1. middle colic artery
2. right colic artery
3. marginal artery
4. ileocolic artery
5. ascending colon
6. caecal arteries
7. ileum (cut)
8. caecum
9. transverse mesocolon
10. transverse colon (displaced)
11. pancreas
12. superior mesenteric vein
13. jejunal arteries (cut)
14. mesentery of small intestine (cut)
15. ileal arteries (cut)
16. appendix & mesoappendix
17. sigmoid colon

Fig. 4.20
1. superior mesenteric vessels (cut)
2. inferior mesenteric vein & artery
3. left ureter
4. sigmoid vessels

5. mesocolon (cut)
6. spleen
7. left colic flexure (cut)
8. inferior pole of left kidney
9. ascending & descending branches of left colic artery
10. descending colon
11. left gonadal vessels

Fig. 4.21
1. spleen
2. liver (cut)
3. gastroduodenal artery (cut)
4. hepatic artery
5. portal vein
6. bile duct
7. duodenum (cut)
8. superior mesenteric vein
9. superior mesenteric artery
10. splenic vein
11. inferior mesenteric vein

Fig. 4.22
1. suprarenal gland
2. superior mesenteric artery (cut)
3. right renal vein
4. psoas major
5. inferior vena cava
6. left renal vein
7. kidney
8. left gonadal vein
9. ureter
10. first lumbar nerve
11. quadratus lumborum

Fig. 4.23
1. hepatic veins (cut)
2. suprarenal gland
3. renal fascia (cut)
4. perirenal fat (cut)
5. psoas major
6. hepatic artery (cut)
7. inferior vena cava
8. renal vein
9. branches of renal artery
10. ureter
11. right gonadal vein

Fig. 4.24
1. right suprarenal artery
2. median arcuate ligament
3. psoas major
4. renal vein (cut)
5. lumbar vein & inferior vena cava
6. right common iliac artery
7. right & left common iliac veins
8. inferior phrenic artery
9. coeliac trunk (cut)
10. renal artery & suprarenal branch
11. superior mesenteric artery (cut)
12. gonadal arteries
13. inferior mesenteric artery
14. lumbar artery
15. bifurcation of aorta

Fig. 4.25
1. hepatic & splenic arteries (cut)
2. aortic lymph nodes
3 inferior vena cava
4. gonadal vein
5. common iliac nodes
6. left gastric artery
7. superior mesenteric artery (cut)
8. right gonad artery (cut)
9. aorta
10. inferior mesenteric artery

Fig. 4.26
1. diaphragm
2. psoas minor tendon & psoas major
3. iliac crest
4. transversus abdominis
5. sympathetic trunk
6 iliacus
7. femoral nerve
8. lumbosacral trunk
9. obturator nerve
10. subcostal nerve
11. quadratus lumborum
12. liohypogastric nerve
13. ilioinguinal nerve
14. iliac & psoas fasciae
15. genitofemoral nerve

Fig. 4.27
1. genitofemoral nerve
2. iliohypogastric nerve
3. ilioinguinal nerve
4. lateral cutaneous nerve of thigh
5. femoral nerve
6. obturator nerve
7. lumbosacral trunk

Fig. 4.28
1. central tendon
2. inferior vena cava (cut)
3. right crus
4 medial arcuate ligament
5. sympathetic trunk
6. subcostal nerve
7. inferior phrenic vein
8. oesophagus (cut)
9. inferior phrenic arteries
10. median arcuate ligament
11. abdominal aorta (cut)
12. vertebrocostal trigone

Chapter 5   Pelvis & Perineum

Fig. 5.1
1. common iliac artery
2. external iliac artery
3. obturator artery entering obturator canal
4. sacrospinous ligament
5. internal iliac artery
6. arteries to pelvic organs
7. artery to gluteal region entering greater sciatic foramen
8. internal pudendal artery

Fig. 5.2
1. uterine tube
2. rectouterine pouch

3. fundus of uterus
4. ovary
5. sigmoid colon (cut)
6. broad ligament
7. vesicouterine pouch
8 bladder

Fig. 5.3
1. cervix
2. bladder
3. fundus
4. uterine cavity
5. body
6. cervical canal
7. posterior fornix
8. external os
9. vesicouterine pouch
10. anterior fornix
11. vagina

Fig. 5.4
1. uterine tube
2. ovary
3. round ligament of uterus
4. uterine vein & artery
5. rectum
6. ovarian vessels
7. ureter
8. internal iliac artery & vein
9. superior rectal vessels (cut)
10. obturator artery
11. obturator nerve
12. rectouterine pouch

Fig. 5.5
1. rectum (cut)
2. levator ani
3. vagina (cut)
4. internal urethral meatus
5. urethra
6. pubic symphysis

Fig. 5.6
1. bladder
2. puboprostatic ligaments
3. prostatic urethra
4. membranous urethra
5. intrabulbar fossa
6. corpus spongiosum
7. spongy urethra
8. glans penis
9. prostate gland
10. bulb of penis
11. navicular fossa

Fig. 5.7
1. ureter
2. vas deferens & ampulla
3 obturator internus
4. posterior surface of bladder
5. prostate
6. left seminal vesicle
7. ischial spine

Fig. 5.8
1 abnormal obturator artery
2. bladder
3. internal iliac artery
4. ureter
5. obturator nerve
6. vas deferens
7. pelvic plexus
8. obturator vein

9. seminal vesicle
10. rectum

Fig. 5.9
1. obturator internus
2 rectum (opened)
3. levator ani
4. anal canal
5. fat in ischiorectal fossa
6. ischial tuberosity
7 perianal skin

Fig. 5.10
1. corpus spongiosum
2. corpus cavernosum
3. bulbospongiosus (cut)
4. crus
5. bulb
6 superficial transverse perineal muscle (cut)
7. external anal sphincter
8. spermatic cord (cut)
9. ischiocavernosus
10. ischial ramus
11. perineal membrane

Fig. 5.11
1. prepuce (cut)
2 ischiocavernosus
3. bulbospongiosus
4. vaginal opening
5. greater vestibular gland
6. ramus of pubis & body
7 crus
8. glans & shaft of clitoris
9. perineal membrane
10. bulb of vestibule (cut)
11. external urethral meatus

Chapter 6   Lower Limb

Fig. 6.1
1. hip bone
2. sacrum
3. femur
4. patella
5. tibia
6. fibula
7. tarsals
8. metatarsals
9. phalanges

Fig. 6.2
1. aorta
2. common iliac
3. superior & inferior gluteal
4. internal iliac
5. linguinal ligament
6. external iliac
7. medial & lateral circumflex femoral
8. femoral
9. obturator
10. profunda femoris with perforating branches
11. popliteal
12. posterior tibial
13. anterior tibial
14. peroneal
15. lateral plantar
16. dorsalis pedis
17. plantar arch
18. medial plantar

Answers

Fig. 6.3
1. sciatic
2. femoral
3. obturator
4. tibial
5. common peroneal
6. deep & superficial peroneal
7. medial & lateral plantar

Fig. 6.4
1. iliopsoas
2. tensor fasciae latae
3. pectineus
4. sartorius
5. adductor longus
6. rectus femoris
7. gracilis
8. vastus lateralis & medialis
9. iliotibial tract

Fig. 6.5
1. lateral cutaneous nerve of thigh
2. iliopsoas
3. femoral nerve
4. lateral circumflex femoral artery
5. sartorius
6. nerve to vastus medialis
7. vastus medialis
8. superficial inguinal ring
9. pectineus
10. adductor longus
11. femoral vein
12. saphenous nerve
13. adductor magnus
14. gracilis

Fig. 6.6
1. pectineus (cut)
2. superior pubic ramus
3. obturator externus
4. anterior & posterior divisions of obturator nerve
5. pectineus (cut)
6. adductor brevis
7. adductor magnus
8. gracilis
9. quadriceps femoris

Fig. 6.7
1. iliopsoas (cut)
2. anterior & posterior divisions of obturator nerve (cut)
3. psoas bursa
4. capsule of hip joint
5. obturator externus
6. iliopsoas (cut)
7. adductor magnus (cut)
8. sciatic nerve
9. hamstrings
10. adductor magnus (cut)
11. gracilis

Fig. 6.8
1. superior gluteal artery
2. inferior gluteal nerve
3. sciatic nerve
4. posterior cutaneous nerve of thigh
5. iliac crest

Fig. 6.8 (cont)
6. gluteus maximus
7. gluteus medius
8. piriformis
9. inferior gluteal artery
10. greater trochanter
11. fascia lata (cut)
12. iliotibial tract
13. attachment of gluteus maximus to gluteal tuberosity

Fig. 6.9
1. pudendal nerve
2. nerve to obturator internus
3. sacrotuberous ligament
4. posterior cutaneous nerve of thigh
5. inferior gluteal vessels & nerves
6. piriformis
7. obturator internus tendon & gemelli
8. nerve to quadratus femoris
9. gluteus maximus
10. quadratus femoris
11. internal pudendal artery
12. adductor magnus
13. sciatic nerve

Fig. 6.10
1. sciatic nerve
2. attachment of gluteus maximus to gluteal tuberosity
3. ischial tuberosity
4. branches to hamstrings
5. long head of biceps femoris
6. semimembranosus
7. branch to short head
8. short head of biceps femoris
9. popliteal artery & vein
10. semitendinosus
11. tibial nerve
12. common peroneal nerve
13. medial & lateral head of gastrocnemius

Fig. 6.11
1. popliteal vein traversing opening in adductor magnus
2. popliteal artery
3. semimembranosus
4. semitendinosus
5. muscular branches
6. tibial nerve
7. biceps femoris
8. lateral head of gastrocnemius
9. common peroneal nerve
10. medial head of gastrocnemius

Fig. 6.12
1. popliteal artery
2. heads of gastrocnemius (reflected)
3. popliteal vein
4. plantaris
5. tibial nerve
6. soleus
7. soleal arch

Fig. 6.12 (cont)
8. tendon of plantaris
9. gastrocnemius (cut)

Fig. 6.13
1. tibialis posterior
2. posterior tibial artery
3. peroneal artery
4. tibial nerve
5. flexor digitorum longus
6. flexor retinaculum
7. soleus
8. fibula
9. flexor hallucis longus
10. tendon of tibialis posterior
11. tendo calcaneum

Fig. 6.14
1. tendon of flexor digitorum longus
2. tibialis posterior attachment
3. tibial nerve
4. tendon of flexor hallucis longus
5. tendon of flexor digitorum longus
6. lateral plantar nerve & artery
7. posterior tibial artery
8. tendon of tibialis posterior
9. tendon of flexor hallucis longus
10. tendo calcaneus (cut)
11. flexor retinaculum
12. abductor hallucis (cut)
13. medial plantar artery & nerve

Fig. 6.15
1. fibrous flexor sheaths
2. branches of lateral plantar nerve
3. abductor digiti minimi
4. flexor digitorum brevis
5. edges of intermuscular septa
6. tendon of flexor digitorum longus
7. tendon of flexor digitorum brevis
8. lumbrical
9. branches of medial plantar nerve
10. abductor hallucis
11. plantor aponeurosis (cut)

Fig. 6.16
1. tendon of flexor digitorum longus
2. medial plantar artery
3. abductor hallucis
4. abductor digiti minimi
5. tendon of flexor hallucis longus
6. plantar metatarsal artery
7. lumbricals
8. heads of flexor hallucis brevis
9. flexor accessorius
10. lateral plantar artery
11. medial & lateral plantar nerves (cut)
12. flexor digitorum brevis (cut)

Fig. 6.17
1. plantar metatarsal arteries
2. deep transverse metatarsal ligament
3. plantar interosseous muscles
4. dorsal interosseous muscles
5. plantar arch
6. adductor hallucis (cut)
7. lateral & medial plantar arteries

Fig. 6.18
1. adductor hallucis oblique head (cut)
2. base of fifth metatarsal
3. tendon of peroneus brevis
4. tendon of peroneus longus
5. long plantar ligament
6. anterior tubercle of calcaneum
7. flexor hallucis longus (cut)
8. base of first metatarsal
9. tendon of tibialis anterior
10. tendon of tibialis posterior & slips
11. flexor retinaculum
12. tendon of flexor digitorum longus (cut)
13. posterior tibial artery (cut)
14. tibial nerve (cut)

Fig. 6.19
1. peroneus longus
2. tibialis anterior
3. subcutaneous surface of tibia
4. extensor digitorum longus
5. peroneus brevis
6. superficial peroneal nerve (cut)
7. peroneus tertius
8. extensor retinaculum
9. tendons of extensor digitorum longus
10. tendon of extensor hallucis longus
11. tendon of tibialis anterior
12. extensor digitorum brevis
13. tendon of peroneus tertius
14. dorsalis pedis artery
15. sural nerve
16. tendons of extensor digitorum brevis

Fig. 6.20
1. common peroneal nerve
2. peroneus longus (reflected)
3. neck of fibula
4. peroneus longus (cut)
5. superficial peroneal nerve (cut)
6. peroneus brevis
7. lateral malleolus
8. extensor digitorum brevis
9. anterior tibial artery
10. extensor digitorum longus (cut)
11. interosseous membrane
12. deep peroneal nerve

99

13. extensor digitorum
    longus (cut)
14. tibialis anterior
15. extensor hallucis longus
16. anterior tibial artery
17. deep peroneal nerve

Fig. 6.21
1. iliopsoas (cut)
2. gluteus maximus
3. iliofemoral ligament
4. pubofemoral ligament
5. psoas tendon (cut)
6. adductor magnus
7. rectus femoris
8. inguinal ligament
9. femoral nerve & vessels
10. femoral canal
11. superior pubic ramus
12. obturator nerve (cut)
13. psoas bursa (opened)
14. obturator externus

Fig. 6.22
1. acetabular labrum
2. gluteal muscles
3. neck of femur
4. articular cartilage
5. ligamentum teres
6. obturator internus &
   externus
7. vastus lateralis
8. iliacus & psoas
9. external iliac vein &
   artery
10. internal iliac artery
11. femoral nerve
12. obturator membrane
13. ischial ramus
14. adductor muscles

Fig. 6.23
1. quadriceps tendon
2. suprapatellar bursa
3. patella
4. infrapatellar fat pad
5. ligamentum patellae
6. meniscus
7. tibial tubercle
8. vastus intermedius
9. hamstring muscles
10. popliteal artery & vein
11. fat
12. gastrocnemius
13. capsule
14. popliteus

Fig. 6.24
1. medial collateral ligament
2. posterior cruciate
   ligament
3. medial meniscus
4. lateral & medial tibial
   condyles
5. lateral meniscus
6. popliteus (cut)
7. tibialis posterior
8. line of attachment of
   capsule
9. medial femoral condyle
10. lateral collateral ligament
11. lateral femoral condyle
12. anterior cruciate
    ligament
13. popliteus tendon (cut)

14. proximal tibiofibular
    joint (opened)
15. anterior tibial artery

Fig. 6.25
1. flexor hallucis longus
2. tendo calcaneus (cut)
3. joint capsule
4. calcaneofibular ligament
5. talus
6. anterior talofibular
   ligament
7. capsule (cut)
8. lateral malleolus
9. extensor digitorum brevis
10. subtalar joint
11. peroneus longus & brevis
    tendons
12. posterior talofibular
    ligament
13. calcaneum

Fig. 6.26
1. great saphenous vein
2. tendon of tibialis anterior
3. tibia
4. tendons of tibialis
   posterior & flexor
   digitorum longus
5. posterior tibial nerve &
   artery
6. lateral malleolus
7. deep peroneal nerve
8. tendon of extensor
   digitorum longus
9. anterior tibial artery with
   venae comitantes
10. tendon of extensor
    hallucis longus
11. tendons of peroneus
    longus & brevis
12. sural nerve
13. short saphenous vein
14. tendon of flexor hallucis
    longus
15. tendo calcaneus

Fig. 6.27
1. tibia
2. head of talus
3. medial cuneiform
4. head of first metatarsal
5. sesamoid bone
6. tendon of extensor
   hallucis longus
7. tendon of flexor hallucis
   longus
8. interosseous talocalcaneal
   ligament
9. sustentaculum tali
10. calcaneum
11. navicular
12. plantar calcaneonavicular
    ligament
13. plantar aponeurosis
14. intrinsic muscles

Chapter 7   Head & Neck
Fig. 7.1
1. maxillary artery
2. facial artery
3. lingual artery
4. external carotid artery
5. common carotid artery

6. superficial temporal
   artery
7. occipital artery
8. internal carotid artery
9. vertebral artery

Fig. 7.2
1. maxillary vein
2. facial vein
3. anterior jugular vein
4. superficial temporal vein
5. retromandibular vein
6. external jugular vein
7. vertebral vein
8. internal jugular vein

Fig. 7.3
1. investing fascia
2. pretracheal fascia
3. carotid sheath
4. prevertebral fascia

Fig. 7.4
1. sternomastoid
2. investing fascia
3. trapezius
4. submandibular gland

Fig. 7.5
1. prevertebral muscles
2. vertebral artery
3. spinal cord
4. postvertebral muscles
5. prevertebral fascia

Fig. 7.6
1. pretrachial fascia
2. larynx & pharynx
3. vagus nerve
4. external carotid artery
5. carotid sheath
6. internal carotid artery
7. internal jugular vein

Fig. 7.7
1. levator scapulae
2. scalenus medius
3. inferior belly of
   omohyoid
4. scalenus anterior
5. nerve to subclavius
6. splenius capitis
7. dorsal scapular nerve
8. scalenus posterior
9. long thoracic nerve
10. parts of brachial plexus
11. suprascapular nerve

Fig. 7.8
1. great auricular nerve
2. transverse cervical nerve
3. anterior jugular vein
4. suprascapular artery
5. subclavian vein
6. external jugular vein
7. lesser occipital nerve
8. spinal accessory nerve
9. proprioceptive fibres for
   trapezius
10. supraclavicular nerves
11. transverse cervical artery
12. inferior belly of
    omohyoid

Fig. 7.9
1. pyramidal lobe

2. cricothyroid
3. middle thyroid vein
4. inferior thyroid veins
5. superior thyroid artery
6. superior thyroid vein
7. left lateral lobe of thyroid
   gland
8. internal jugular vein
9. isthmus
10. common carotid artery

Fig. 7.10
1. common carotid artery
2. trachea
3. internal jugular vein
4. vagus nerve
5. inferior thyroid veins
6. left brachiocephalic vein
7. thyrocervical trunk
8. vagus nerve
9. scalenus anterior
10. phrenic nerve
11. brachial plexus
12. subclavian vein & artery
13. thoracic duct
14. subclavius

Fig. 7.11
1. maxillary artery
2. external carotid artery
3. stylohyoid
4. facial artery
5. lingual artery
6. external carotid artery
7. superior thyroid artery
8. transverse facial artery
9. superficial temporal
   artery
10. internal jugular vein (cut)
11. sternomastoid (cut)
12. posterior auricular artery
    (cut)
13. accessory nerve
14. occipital artery
15. hypoglossal nerve
16. internal carotid artery
17. carotid sinus
18. vagus nerve

Fig. 7.12
1. frontalis
2. orbital & palpebral parts
   of orbicularis oculi
3. levator labii superioris
   alaeque nasi
4. levator anguli oris
5. orbicularis oris
6. depressor labii inferioris
7. mentalis
8. epicranial aponeurosis
9. compressor nares
10. levator labii superioris
11. zygomaticus major &
    minor
12. buccinator
13. risorius
14. depressor anguli oris
15. platysma

Fig. 7.13
1. temporalis
2. zygomatic arch (cut)
3. coronoid process
4. external acoustic meatus
5. capsule of temporo-
   mandibular joint

6. ramus of mandible
7. angle of mandible

Fig. 7.14
1. coronoid process
2. mylohyoid line
3. mental foramen
4. head
5. neck
6. mandibular canal
7. lingula
8. angle

Fig. 7.15
1. deep temporal nerve
2. nerve to upper head of lateral pterygoid
3. buccal nerve
4. lingual nerve
5. inferior alveolar artery & nerve
6. middle meningeal artery
7. auriculotemporal nerve
8. medial pterygoid
9. chorda tympani

Fig. 7.16
1. inferior alveolar nerve
2. lingual nerve
3. nerve to mylohyoid
4. styloglossus
5. stylohyoid
6. anterior belly of digastric
7. nerve to thyrohyoid
8. maxillary artery (cut)
9. styloid process
10. posterior belly of digastric
11. sternomastoid
12. external carotid artery (cut)
13. facial artery
14. hypoglossal nerve
15. lingual artery

Fig. 7.17
1. lingual nerve
2. submandibular duct
3. genioglossus
4. mandible
5. geniohyoid
6. hypoglossal nerve (cut)
7. hyoglossus (cut)
8. stylopharyngeus
9. ascending palatine artery
10. glossopharyngeal nerve
11. tonsillar artery
12. facial artery
13. lingual artery

Fig. 7.18
1. hard palate
2. genioglossus
3. mandible
4. geniohyoid
5. mylohyoid
6. longitudinal intrinsic muscle fibres
7. oropharynx
8. epiglottis
9. hyoid bone

Fig. 7.19
1. frontal lobe
2. orbit
3. maxillary air sinus

4. alveolar ridge
5. nasal septum
6. ethmoidal air cells
7. middle concha
8. middle meatus
9. inferior concha
10. hard palate
11. mandible
12. genioglossus

Fig. 7.20
1. olfactory bulb & nerves
2. sphenoidal air sinus
3. auditory tube
4. hard palate
5. cribriform plate
6. superior concha
7. middle concha
8. vestibule
9. inferior concha

Fig. 7.21
1. pharyngeal tonsil
2. auditory tube
3. nasopharynx
4. soft palate
5. palatopharyngeal ridge
6. oropharynx
7. epiglottis
8. laryngopharynx
9. cricoid cartilage
10. nasal cavity
11. hard palate
12. oral cavity
13. palatoglossal ridge
14. palatine tonsil
15. mandible
16. tongue
17. hyoid bone
18. thyroid cartilage
19. laryngeal cavity

Fig. 7.22
1. internal jugular vein
2. internal carotid artery
3. superior, middle & inferior constrictors
4. cervical sympathetic trunk
5. vagus nerve
6. pharyngeal raphe
7. ascending pharyngeal artery
8. vagus nerve & pharyngeal branch
9. superior laryngeal nerve
10. pharyngeal plexus
11. thyroid gland
12. common carotid & subclavian arteries
13. recurrent laryngeal nerve

Fig. 7.23
1. greater horn of hyoid bone
2. aryepiglottic muscle
3. cricothyroid articulation
4. recurrent laryngeal nerve
5. superior horn of thyroid cartilage
6. interarytenoid muscle
7. posterior cricoarytenoid
8. cricoid lamina

Fig. 7.24
1. mucous membrane

2. interarytenoid
3. cricoid lamina
4. trachea
5. hyoid
6. epiglottic cartilage
7. thyroid cartilage
8. vestibular fold
9. saccule
10. vocal fold
11. cricoid arch
12. first tracheal ring

Fig. 7.25
1. coronal suture
2. greater wing
3. lateral pterygoid plate
4. pterygoid hamulus
5. external acoustic meatus
6. lambdoid suture
7. styloid process
8. mastoid process
9. zygomatic process

Fig. 7.26
1. superior sagittal sinus
2. straight sinus
3. dura
4. falx cerebri
5. cerebral hemisphere
6. tentorium cerebelli
7. transverse sinus
8. cerebellum

Fig. 7.27
1. internal carotid artery
2. oculomotor (III) nerve
3. trigeminal (V) nerve
4. abducens (VI) nerve
5. facial (VII) & vestibulocochlear (VIII) nerves
6. glossopharyngeal (IX), vagus (X) & accessory (XI) nerves
7. optic chiasma
8. ophthalmic (Va) & maxillary (Vb) divisions
9. left posterior cerebral artery
10. mandibular (Vc) division
11. trigeminal ganglion
12. motor root
13. trochlear (IV) nerve
14. hypoglossal (XII) nerve

Fig. 7.28
1. supraorbital nerve
2. levator palpebrae superioris
3. frontal nerve
4. lacrimal nerve
5. supratrochlear nerve
6. trochlea
7. superior oblique
8. superior rectus
9. trochlear (IV) nerve

Fig. 7.29
1. levator palpebrae superioris (cut)
2. superior oblique tendon
3. superior rectus (cut)
4. lacrimal gland
5. long ciliary nerve
6. short ciliary nerves
7. superior division of

oculomotor (III) nerve (cut)
8. superior rectus (cut)
9. trochlea
10. superior oblique
11. ophthalmic artery
12. optic (II) nerve
13. posterior ethmoidal nerve
14. nasociliary nerve
15. trochlear (IV) nerve
16. levator palpebrae superioris (cut)
17. frontal nerve (cut)
18. optic (II) nerve

Chapter 8   Back

Fig. 8.1
1. transversospinalis
2. transverse process
3. tubercle of rib
4. shaft of rib
5. spinous process
6. trapezius
7. head of rib
8. superior articular facet
9. erector spinae
10. serratus posterior
11. latissimus dorsi

Fig. 8.2
1. vertebral body
2. foramen transversarium
3. spinal cord
4. superior articular facet
5. anterior median fissure
6. vertebral foramen
7. ventral root
8. ventral ramus
9. spinal nerve
10. dorsal ramus
11. dorsal root & ganglion
12. medial & lateral branches

Fig. 8.3
1. anterior tubercle
2. posterior tubercle
3. body
4. superior articular process
5. foramen transversarium
6. spinous process
7. lamina
8. inferior articular process

Fig. 8.4
1. lamina
2. vertebral foramen
3. body
4. foramen transversarium
5. superior articular facet
6. anterior tubercle
7. bifid spine
8. pedicle
9. posterior tubercle

Fig. 8.5
1. occipital bone
2. atlanto-occipital joint
3. posterior arch of atlas
4. lateral atlantoaxial joint
5. occipital condyle
6. styloid process
7. transverse process of atlas
8. dens

9. spinous process of axis
10. body of axis

Fig. 8.6
1. costal facets
2. body
3. spinous process
4. superior articular process
5. inferior intervertebral notch
6   inferior articular process

Fig. 8.7
1. lamina
2. body
3. superior anticular process
4. transverse process
5. spinous process
6. pedicle

Fig. 8.8
1. pedicle
2. body

3. superior articular process
4. transverse process
5. spinous process
6. inferior articular facet

Fig. 8.9
1. superior articular facet
2. body
3. pedicle
4. transverse process
5. spinous process
6. vertebral foramen
7. lamina

Fig. 8.10
1. lumbar vertebral body
2. anterior longitudinal ligament
3. lumbar spinal nerve in intervertebral foramen
4. intervertebral disc
5. pedicle

Fig. 8.11
1. splenius
2. pinna
3. sternomastoid
4. longissimus
5. iliocostalis
6. external intercostal muscles
7. ribs
8. external abdominal oblique
9. position of iliac crest

Fig. 8.12
1. spinal cord
2. pia
3. transverse process
4. anterior median fissure
5. subarachnoid space
6. arachnoid
7. extradural space
8. dura
9. spinous process

Fig. 8.13
1. vertebral body
2. psoas major
3. hilum of kidney
4. kidney
5. quadratus lumborum
6. inferior articular process of LI
7. liver
8. cauda equina
9. kidney
10. erector spinae
11. transversospinalis
12. conus

Index